I0420728

AUTOPHAGY FOR WOMEN

EXTENDED AND INTERMITTENT WATER FASTING
IS THE POWERFUL SECRET OF ANTI-AGING AND
REJUVENATION USING YOUR BODY'S INNATE
INTELLIGENCE

DANA WELLS

Copyright © 2019 by Dana Wells

All rights reserved.

No part of this book may be reproduced in any form or by any electronic or mechanical means, including information storage and retrieval systems, without written permission from the author, except for the use of brief quotations in a book review.

Being a healthy woman isn't about getting on a scale or measuring your waistline. We need to start focusing on what matters - on how we feel, and how we feel about ourselves

— MICHELLE OBAMA

AUTOPHAGY FOR WOMEN

CONTENTS

DISCLAIMER

This book is not intended to replace medical advice. It is not responsible for the actions and results of the reader. Please seek out the advice of a doctor before starting any health program. The author is not a medical doctor, and the information in this book is meant to supplement your health changes, not dictate them. The wonders of autophagy are still being discovered as this book was written. Please enjoy this information we provide but also be wise in consuming it.

INTRODUCTION

Congratulations on downloading *Autophagy for Women* and thank you for doing so.

The following chapters will discuss the important role that autophagy plays in the health and performance of our bodies down to the cellular level. Find out how critical this process is in determining metabolic rate, cellular lifespan, recycling materials, and keeping the cells in a clean and supportive environment. Autophagy also determines how much fat your body burns for fuel. Autophagy is a natural process in the body that is rarely talked about, yet seems to hold an important position in cellular management.

This book will discuss both the history of autophagy discoveries and the importance to your overall health and other benefits. Learn what triggers autophagy and how it can be used to your advantage. Find out why it's the most effective tool you can have for increased energy, anti-aging, weight management, weight loss, boosting immunity, and more.

Find out who can benefit the most from autophagy and how it can turn the clock back in renewing energy and help prevent neurode-generative diseases like Parkinson's, Alzheimer's, and early-onset dementia. Learning how to trigger autophagy can change your life and transform the lives of those around you. Imagine having the knowledge to help prevent these terrible diseases at your fingertips.

Discover how an intermittent and extended water fast can accelerate the autophagy process. Find out how to try these fasts and experience the benefits yourself. You'll get the complete guide to preparing and doing each fast quickly, as well as the warning signs for any problems. All the science is understandable, and you'll love how easy the process will be.

There are plenty of books on this subject on the market, so thanks again for choosing this one! Every effort was made to ensure it is full of as much useful information as possible. Please enjoy!

WHAT IS AUTOPHAGY?

Autophagy or *autophagocytosis* is a Greek word that literally translates to "self-eating." It's a natural cellular process that allows for the sorting through, recycling, or getting rid of cell parts, pieces, or dead and dying cells that are regulated by the body. Autophagy can happen naturally or be induced by special methods. It is one of the deepest, lasting body cleanses you can undergo since it happens deep at the cellular level. It can seek out items that are harmful or keep your cells getting the right nutrition on a regular basis.

The Science of Autophagy

The human body has the ability to initiate a little-known secret process of clean-up and self-improvement in both a natural and specifically triggered way. Rather than focusing on eating specific foods, the deprivation of food results in boosting this natural process by appreciable amounts. Naturally skipping meals makes the method easy and seem like a normal part of your routine.

Unless you are trying to restrict your calories purposefully, the act of missing meals will make it relatively unnecessary to track your exact caloric intake. You can get very detailed with the process and count everything down to the final calorie. It gives you a great deal of leverage and flexibility when using autophagy to reset your body's health and wellness.

Autophagy and Cellular-Level "Cleaning" or Regeneration

The housekeeping duties within the body that help clear up an accumulation of broken down cells or deformed cellular structures and components are kicked into high gear when autophagy begins. The body will actually digest the dead or defective cells and parts, converting the material into added energy. It's a more selective process than attained during periods of "starvation" that trigger the body to begin eating completing healthy cells for energy and maintenance.

Autophagy sees the overall cells and gathers up the damaged, dysfunctional, and dying cells and cell matter for removal, while leaving the healthy cells alone. It's a regenerative process that increases the stability of the organs and tissues throughout the body. The natural ability to do this lessens over time. It means that activating autophagy can bring your body back into a more youthful state, at least at the cellular operational levels. No special foods or chemical mixtures are required.

Innate Intelligence and Sorting the Good and Bad

How does the body know how to separate out the harmful or useless stuff from the good? The cellular operations of the body work with intelligence and purpose. All the cells and loose cellular materials are scoured and evaluated for condition, function, and completeness. Anything that doesn't match up with a good cellular profile is digested and converted to energy. It keeps the body clear of a buildup in material that is non-productive and possibly harmful. It clears the way for the body to multiply healthy cells and tissues.

The great thing about these innate intelligent operations is that they require no thought or cognitive understanding on your part in order to work. You don't have to think, plan, or worry about whether your body is doing this on a routine basis. Once the conditions are met, autophagy happens. It's a process that relieves stress in your body from the molecular level.

Natural and Triggered Autophagy

Natural autophagy happens no matter your diet, activity level, or genetic makeup. The problem with natural processes is that they can be hampered by illness, disease, or a simple lack of proper sleep. Slow metabolism and obesity can slow down the cellular cleanup and leave you operating in a less than optimal condition.

You have the ability to speed this process up and induce it on a more frequent basis. Autophagy can be triggered in three different ways.

Regular Exercise:

Regular, rigorous exercise does enough damage to the cells of your muscles to trigger autophagy in an attempt to move the damaged cells out and allow new cells to grow. The rate and amount of exercise needed to initiate this response is unknown. You can feel a sudden surge of fresh energy directly after a workout. The cleansing brought about at the cellular level is somewhat responsible.

Lower Carb Intake:

Lowering your intake of carbohydrates is another viable method of triggering autophagy in women. Carbs and sugars are turned into immediate energy to be used by the body. Eating diets with a stronger focus on increased proteins and fats, with fewer carbs and sugar results in the body beginning to "eat" the existing fat reserves to obtain energy. The "cannibalism" action is, by definition, autophagy.

Fasting:

The act of going periods of time without food routinely is called fasting. Although this book will only focus on extended and intermittent water fasting, there are a variety of different methods. The results of fasting are triggering a deeper body cleansing by autophagy than any other method known. You can begin using autophagy as a tool to clear up damaged or diseased cells throughout the body completely.

The Recognition of Autophagy

The first notable observation and recognition of autophagy was by a man named Keith Porter in 1962 at the Rockefeller Institute. The recognition of lysosomes with mitochondria in rat liver cells after adding glucagon was wrongly thought to be the observation of developing lysosomes. It would be decades before autophagy-related cells were given prominence in the study of yeast.

The Breakthrough of Autophagy

The 1990s saw a great expansion of research and knowledge of autophagy and how it could benefit people. Beth Levine and her research group learned of the connections of autophagy and cancer in 1999. It has since expanded to benefits in the corrections of neurodegeneration and immune system defense. Solid evidence-based research proved that starvation-induced autophagy cleansed the body of parts and pieces of cells and cellular material.

Nobel Prize-Worthy Discovery

In 2016, the Nobel Prize in physiology/medicine was awarded to Yoshinori Ohsumi for determining the autophagy gene with a specified protocol. It has stirred and renewed commitment to researching the connections of the naturally triggered cleansing action of genes in the human body.

Some debate surrounded the awarding of the Nobel Prize to one individual for what was viewed as collective work by many parties, but the benefits are far-reaching past the accolades. It set the wheels in motion towards devising actual treatments to initiate autophagy to see the impact in the battle against some devastating diseases and troubling genetic abnormalities.

Using Natural Cell Selection to Better Your Health

The process of fasting has been done for centuries, in one form or another. The one consistent feature that has kept the activity popular is the shared belief that you feel better and healthier afterward. Science has since proven that fasting does trigger autophagy, which sets the cells of the body in motion to clean things up a little bit. The use of autophagy to target the removal of harmful, or at least non-helpful matter from the body leads to better overall health. No other outcome can reasonably be expected.

Viruses and Diseased Cells

The old mantra "starve a fever and feed a cold" has some grounding in fact, so it seems. Autophagy can and will target viruses and cells that exhibit abnormal growth, such as cancer or other cellular degenerative conditions. Getting rid of these things can quickly accelerate your recovery.

The old myth that eating during high fever took attention away from fighting the illness and put efforts towards digestion was false. Periods of fasting, when sickened with a virus, helped concentrate efforts by the body to get rid of whatever was unnatural, unhelpful, and flat-out harmful.

Dead and Dying Cells

The programmed life and death of your cells ensure that cyclical cell die-offs and regeneration happen throughout your body at designated times. Everything is programmed to do this at acceptable intervals to avoid catastrophe. Natural autophagy is triggered during this process and helps eliminate the dead and dying cells. As you age, the process slows appreciably.

Artificially triggering autophagy is a way to make up for the slowing of regeneration with age and give your body a more youthful, invigorating burst of cellular level cleansing. You will notice differences that are more than skin deep. The energy you feel will be more consistent, and your overall power will increase. Slow and sluggish cellular activity can impact every area of your body and hinder your performance mentally, as well as physically.

Cell Clutter and Debris

Cell damage, regardless of the reasons, will leave behind debris and clutter like mitochondria. Getting rid of this clutter is done easily with autophagy. Initiating autophagy through exercise was tested through the Beth Levine Group in the 1990s. It proved unhelpful when it came to clearing out already existing cellular debris and clutter. In fact, it created more debris from the damage to tissues that exercise normally creates.

It was discovered that initiating or triggering autophagy AFTER exercise is where the real clean-up took place. It happens on a grand scale, leaving nothing behind that was not beneficial for the cells and body, as a whole. Maintaining muscle homeostasis during exercise, especially with collagen fibers, benefits greatly from a phase of autophagy between exercise routines.

Targeted Autophagy

Developing methods of therapeutic autophagy for cancer was the goal of all the work done by the Beth Levine Group. Discovering ways to use the natural abilities to nourish or deprive particular cells could pave the way for guaranteed treatment of a disease that claims millions of lives annually. What was learned showed both some promise, but with a few risks thrown in for good measure.

The autophagy process has the ability to cleanse the cells and interstitial spaces so well that almost any type of cell flourishes, including tumors. Inhibiting autophagy is a way of depriving these cells of the necessary nutrients and ridding of waste, causing apoptosis or necrosis.

The second method of utilizing the natural tumor suppression of autophagy allowed for triggering of this state with the hopes of having the tumor dealt with quickly. It has shown some promise in routine treatment for cancer but can backfire and cause the tumor cells to thrive.

Neurodegenerative conditions like Parkinson's disease are greatly improved by the initiation of autophagy, which provides future hope for anyone suffering from nerve-related diseases and conditions that are difficult to trace and treat. More is learned every year in how to use a variety of therapies by triggering or suppressing the autophagy process.

2

BENEFITS OF AUTOPHAGY

THE KNOWN POSITIVE RESULTS BROUGHT ABOUT BY AUTOPHAGY ARE numerous, and research continues to uncover more each year. The process gives a better understanding of how the cells of the body determine what needs to be disposed of, and what can be saved and used again. The helpful nature in managing the internal environment in a way that is beneficial to healthy cellular activity is undeniable. The following list of benefits is not exhaustive, and you will find plenty of good things to be had by pushing for autophagy in your own body. You can finally begin to enjoy a life with less pain, illness, and enjoy youthful energy levels once again.

Autophagy and Aging

A popular perk that comes along with autophagy is winning the battle against aging, even if it's in small ways and measures. You can literally help turn back the pages of time at the cellular level with the right autophagy initiating routines. It's one piece of the puzzle that forms the complete picture of a healthier, more vibrant you.

Improved Brain Function:

The consistent removal of degraded proteins helps you combat the risk of degenerative neurological disorders like Alzheimer's, Parkinson's, and dementia, which strike the aging woman with greater frequency. Autophagy will help sweep out these proteins and improve overall brain function and mental acuity. Concentration, focus, and memory are all positively affected by the autophagy process.

Increased Energy:

Bright, shiny, new healthy cells replace ones that are damaged from stress like exercise or natural cell death. The cleanup period after exercise is one example of how your energy levels are boosted to a new level. Rather than being completely exhausted, you feel ready to take on the world. It's a youthful cellular rejuvenation brought to you, courtesy of autophagy.

Reduce Metabolic Dysfunction:

Diabetes and obesity are better controlled by improving natural metabolic functions. Switching to a lower carb and sugar diet will allow the cells to begin breaking down body fats for energy. It's a natural way to begin shedding extra pounds. Reducing obesity will reduce your chances of diabetes and can correct diabetes type 2. Metabolism slows as you age, and autophagy can help fire it back up to youthful levels.

Inflammation Regulation:

The cells of your body do get inflamed when they are fighting off invading microorganisms that lead to illness or disease. The cells should not STAY in a state of inflammation. When you lack the right amount of autophagy process, the clutter around the cells can lead to a continual inflammation that causes muscles soreness, joint swelling and weakness, and other inflammatory conditions. Autophagy helps regulate the inflammation to promote healthy amounts.

The Basics of Boosting Autophagy:

- Drink green or ginseng tea.
- Eat high anti-oxidant foods like sweet potatoes or cherries.
- Add Omega-3 fatty acids to your diet.
- Cut down on carbohydrates and processed sugars.
- Aerobic Exercise
- Skip snacks and an occasional meal.

These are just a few things you can do on a regular basis to boost your natural autophagy. We will explore deeper triggers in an upcoming chapter. Begin by trying a few of these in combination. Take note of the burst of energy you feel.

Getting Rid of Cellular "Junk"

It's hard to get anything done if the area you have to work with is junked up with items you never use. The cells of your body also experience difficulty operating as they should when debris from damaged or deformed cells builds up. Removing this disposable material is a necessary part of complete physical rejuvenation.

Cellular Stress, Damage, and Debris Trail:

Missing the bus and having to walk to your destination, for miles, unexpectedly, leaves you with muscle soreness in your legs you can feel the next day. Planned activities like moving to a new house, playing in a charity softball game, or a regular workout routine can also "stress" the muscles and cause damage that your body will have to repair.

Cellular stress is not a bad thing. It's required in order to build muscle mass. You work out and cause damage to the tissue. Your body rests and repairs, which leads you to go back and do it all over again. It's the yin and yang of developing stronger, bigger muscles throughout the body, or even in smaller, targeted areas.

Other forms of cellular stress, such as protein deprivation, or fasting, can also work towards speeding up the clean-up autophagy provides. Although there are still ongoing studies, the demonstrable benefits of certain stressors and increased autophagy response show promise in future uses of this method for positive natural cell selection.

Autophagosomes and Natural Cellular-Level Recycling:

Once the cells have determined that cleanup needs to happen, autophagosomes build around the debris materials and every component is sorted, with proteins and other salvageable materials kept and the rest tossed. It's an oversimplification of the chemical and physical processes, but it gives an accurate picture of the ultimate end-result.

Cellular Refreshing:

Anyone that has come off a fast or undergone a heavy-duty physical workout understands the deep level of refreshment felt immediately following the activity. It is mostly attributed to the actions of autophagy in cleaning up the damaged cells and loose debris left in the spaces between your cells. Autophagy also pulls away defective areas of cells, removing anything that's not beneficial to the body. The results are the ability to breathe easier and every area of the body feeling somehow more alive and vibrant.

Improve Metabolism

When it comes to autophagy, not only can it help improve the metabolic rate, but it can change what your body eats to create energy. Anyone can benefit from improved metabolism. You'll feel increased levels of energy, focus, and begin returning to a healthy body weight, if obesity is a problem. You can accomplish all of this without complete starvation or having to exercise several hours a day. No doubt exercise is important, but autophagy allows you to keep it at levels that nearly anyone can handle on a daily basis.

Fats and Carbs:

The energy your body needs can come from a source of stored fat or the more readily available carbohydrate ingestion. Limiting the amounts of carbohydrates through a dietary change or switching to a more ketogenic version forces the body to look for a different source of fuel, which ends up being the fat reserves. It also makes use of the random unusable cellular material and burns it as extra fuel.

The switch to a diet with fewer carbs can be tough if you are a habitual eater of high carbohydrate foods. You should consider making the necessary diet changes that back up autophagy before entering any type of activity that creates cellular stress, such as vigorous exercise or fasting. You can begin the new diet changes months ahead of time and be better prepared for increased levels of autophagy in your body.

Beneficial Redirection of Your Metabolism:

Using autophagy to redirect metabolism and the decisions your cells make to gain energy can be one of the biggest advantages of this process. It can lead to many good things directly tied to an efficient and fast metabolism. One of the immediate benefits is a permanent loss of extra weight.

Reducing levels of obesity can immediately impact your blood sugar levels and rid your body of every symptom of diabetes type

2. Autophagy can also ensure you have a more consistent source of energy your body needs to function well.

Speeding up sluggish metabolism helps bring about a feeling of well-being. You are never completely drained of energy and get more done with less effort during your day. Combined with a cleaner cellular environment, autophagy works to optimize your fat-burning potential for a lifetime of better health.

Reduce Chronic Diseases

Chronic disease is something that ends up placing limits on the lives and lifestyles of all who suffer. It can be due to the levels of pain, swelling, or other symptoms that aren't easily treated. Autophagy can pick out some of the cells that are causing problems and support the natural death of these problematic structures. You can begin a whole new chapter in life that gives you back freedom of movement and freedom from pain.

Cancer:

More and more cell types are being discovered to have everything to do with the sorting and inspection of each cell and inhibiting or helping the growth potential. Cancerous tumors are no exception. Under ideal conditions of limiting autophagy, the inhibition of cancerous cells was observed, but this also happened during some periods of autophagy. It can be expected that increasing autophagy also increases the cellular recognition of unusual cell growth. Although it's far from a cancer cure, it can help by increasing the health of your body to help fight the disease.

Chronic Inflammation:

Chronic inflammation of joints and limbs of the body can make a movement like lifting, gripping, sitting, and standing a painful or difficult task. A lack of proper amount of autophagy is believed to be an associated cause of constant inflammation. The body stays in constant battle-mode to ward off perceived harmful cells like viruses and diseases. Inducing increased levels of autophagy can diminish the constant inflammation and make the body react only when necessary. Removal of cellular "trash" helps this regulate naturally.

Diabetes Type 2

Diabetes is a disease that forces the levels of the hormone called insulin to increase blood sugar in the body. A combination of periodic fasting and reducing carbs or sugars helps diabetes type 2 disappear. Your blood sugar levels will fall off the high-end of the charts and normalize. It requires close monitoring and discussing the idea of fasting with your doctor since some of the medications prescribed for treatment can be affected by fasting. Metformin is one of the medications that have to be taken with food, or at least close to mealtime.

Neurodegenerative disease:

Autophagy seems to improve the neuroplasticity of the brain. Cognitive functions and the ability to think are improved. Memory, concentration, and focus are heightened. Most neurodegenerative conditions improve or are reversed at some level. It's considered an even better way to guard your brain against being affected by neurodegenerative conditions. Say goodbye to the risks of Parkinson's, Alzheimer's, or early-onset dementia.

Increase Cellular Replacement and Youthful Features

The search for the mystical "Fountain of Youth" has taken all sorts of turns and helped push all kinds of products that are supposed to contain the magic formula to regain youth. The answer to aging lies more in the internal workings of the body than any external force you can add or remove. Cellular growth, development, and ability to carry out their designated purpose has everything to do with staying young and feeling great. Autophagy plays an important role in the cells of your body being able to make the most out of the lifespan each is given. Replacing a dying cell faster and more efficiently limits the complications that aging cell activity can bring.

Inviting Environment for Cell Replacement:

Once your body is cleansed of many damaged and random cellular materials, your cells can better determine how to move forward in replacing cells that are aged and dying. Your body will have an easier time conducting the natural cell regenerative process. It's no different from cleaning up a messy room. You feel better and can find the things you need to do more with the space. You can turn back the pages of the calendar to a more youthful cell regeneration ability.

Better Cellular Performance:

The process of autophagy increases the performance of every cell in your body. The recycled materials are put back into play and the rest converted to usable energy to allow cellular operations. All your internal organs, hair, skin, skeleton, and other structures stay in better overall condition. Better cell performance allows the natural process of the body to function well, such as digestion, blood circulation, or nerve stimulation. When every process of your body works in unison, the results are the overwhelming feeling of well-being.

Youthful Look and Feel:

Cellular regeneration is the method your body uses to stay healthy and ensure you have enough new cells to replenish those that are dying off. It's a balancing act that gets harder to manage as the years roll by. The skin begins to lose luster and elasticity. The hair dulls and begins to lose color. The internal organs begin to malfunction. Using deeper states of autophagy is a way to reclaim some of the youthful glow and feel that's lost from poor metabolism and hindered cell regeneration. Over time, other people will begin to notice your increase in energy and exuberance.

Increase Immune System Effectiveness

The immune system of the body is there to help prevent illnesses and quickly heal when you do fall ill. Autophagy works in tandem with your natural immune system to isolate and get rid of cells your body doesn't need. Not every piece of material handled by the autophagy process is a disease or illness causing pathogen, but it's something that is holding your cells back from performing at top levels. Encouraging autophagy is a way to boost your ability to stay healthy and keep your entire body functioning well. Illness will begin to be an isolated problem that you rarely have to tackle.

Determining Good and Bad:

The autophagy state is one that increases the ability of your cells to recognize what is good or bad in all the materials and structures that are close by. Better decisions can be made by your own body on what to keep and what to toss. It requires the cells to have the blueprint handy which is your DNA. It helps keep the DNA in an unaltered or deformed condition. Every part of your body can be replicated with new cells using this specific blueprint.

Removing Pathogens and Useless Materials

Pathogens and harmful materials that hide and linger between the cells can lead to illness and chronic diseases. Autophagy will help find these bits of material, surround them and remove them from the body. It works in a proactive way to prevent you from getting sick, rather than the traditional fighting off illnesses that are given a chance to set up housekeeping. Encouraging autophagy during cold and flu seasons is an extra layer of defense you can provide your body in the bid to stay well.

Encouraging Healthy Production of Brain, Heart, and Organ Cells

The internal organs like the brain, heart, kidneys, liver, and others all begin to undergo a variety of levels of deterioration and degeneration as you age. The brain begins to lose neuroplasticity, and cognitive activities, memory, and concentration become affected. The heart may begin to develop skipped or erratic beating, and the other organs begin to fail at following through with their usual duties. Autophagy is a process in the body that helps rid the system of cells that are not contributing to the proper function of your organs. Instead, healthy vibrant cells are created to replace the dying and deformed ones.

3

HOW TO TRIGGER AUTOPHAGY

TRIGGERING AUTOPHAGY IS A GUARANTEED WAY TO LOSE WEIGHT AND can provide many other health benefits that make you an overall healthier person. Numerous ways exist that allow you to take normal autophagy processes and turn up the volume. The following methods are proven ways to get the full benefits of autophagy in relatively safe ways.

Low-Carb Dieting

Trimming down on the carbohydrates can kick autophagy into high gear. It depends on the level and length of time you restrict the carbs. At some point, the body will switch over and begin eating the stored fat in order to generate the energy needed to sustain life. The stress of potential starvation is what gets the body moving in a direction that is beneficial for anyone wanting a real cleanse or to lose a few pounds. Changing how you look at food is a great first step in being able to tackle huge dietary adjustments.

Ketosis Diet:

The ketosis diet has been popularized by weight lifters worldwide in being able to create lean muscle mass and rid themselves of unwanted fat. Women are fond of this type of diet due to the amount of fat it can take off in a short amount of time. It involves the removal or drastic reduction of carbohydrates and increase in high-fat foods. Carbohydrates are removed like:

- Regular potatoes
- White bread
- Pasta

In its place are sweet potatoes, whole wheat bread, and brown rice. Sweet potatoes are packed with healthy anti-oxidants. Following a complete carb restricted diet can be difficult, but every attempt you make will result in real autophagy benefits.

It's important with a ketosis diet to add high fats that are healthy. 60 to 70 percent of your diet in ketosis should be derived from fats. Choose items like nuts, beans, and lentils to fuel your energy.

Occasional Carbohydrate Restriction:

If you are unwilling or unable to use a strict keto diet plan, try periodic carbohydrate restrictions. Restricting carbs and cutting back drastically on sugary foods and drinks will force the body to begin using the stored fat for food. It does this by boosting autophagy into high-gear. You will begin to notice your clothes are fitting better and women will notice a major loss of inches around the waist. You have successfully tapped into your body's natural way to get to a healthy weight.

Vigorous Exercise

Vigorous exercise is a way to stress the cells and enter a deeper autophagy state. The repair that will be necessary AFTER the exercise is where the benefit of autophagy happens. You'll also get additional benefits of cardio exercise, muscle toning, power building, weight loss, and lowered blood pressure. What kind of exercise would you like to do? A whole world of options is available. Below are only a few suggestions. Keep looking until you find the right one that suits your interests and activity level.

Jogging or Cycling:

Both jogging and cycling can be done in the outdoors or in a stationary setting, such as your home or in a gym. All you need are a good pair of sneakers and a jogging outfit to enjoy these forms of exercise in a gym. You'll need a good bike and safety equipment to cycle in the outdoors.

Aerobics:

Aerobic exercise is great for the heart and blood circulations. It can also burn calories at a fast rate. You can pop in a DVD aerobic training tape and do it from the comfort of home or join a class of like-minded people. You can even start a small group of your own.

Kickboxing:

Kickboxing has become a popular way for women to get a well-rounded form of exercise. It combines the elements of aerobics, martial arts, and other endurance training exercise. Who knows? If you get good enough, you might enter a few competitions. If not, you always have the follow-up benefits of autophagy.

Martial Arts:

The variety of martial arts available to learn and practice are numerous. A few extra benefits of martial arts are the skill developments for self-defense, relaxation techniques, and concentration. You get some well-rounded skills and autophagy-inducing exercise in one activity. Martial arts can be done by DVD instruction at home but is better with private or class instruction.

Swimming:

Swimming is a sport that can involve great cardio exercise, depending on your pace and the length you swim. You can change stroke styles and squeeze more mileage out of each session. It's the perfect sport for hot climates or to combat summertime heat.

Tennis or Racquetball:

Tennis and racquetball will get your heart rate up quickly, especially if you are playing in a competitive fashion. It involves hand-eye coordination, balance, aerobics, and endurance. Tennis can be played outdoors, but racquetball requires an indoor court. Both sports have similar challenges and can be a fun way to pick up your autophagy.

Kayaking:

Getting out on a lake or slow-moving river is a nice way to get a little exercise and enjoy nature. You can test your skills on faster-moving water once you get a little experience under your belt.

Hiking:

The natural terrain of the trail you choose to hike will dictate the difficulty level of this activity. You can adjust your walking speed to bring additional cardio benefits. Take a camera with you to get some pictures or videos of the views you'll enjoy along the way.

No matter what activities or changes you decide to make, keep good nutrition in mind. Low-carb diets are great but don't forget to up the carbs if you are doing exercise or strenuous activity. Nothing replaces a good, wholesome, balanced diet. Reducing sugars and processed foods will provide less cell debris for autophagy to have to clean out.

How Fasting Starts the Autophagy Process

Autophagy is a natural process that happens quietly in the background all the time. Fasting is a trigger that can increase autophagy activity by leaps and bounds. It's difficult to test in humans but has been observed in rats and other animals in laboratory settings. Although the amount of autophagy to expect is relatively unknown, results are always a guarantee with the right triggering conditions.

Nutrition Deprivation and Cellular Stress:

The purposeful depriving of the body of food causes stress to the system that triggers the autophagy process. The cells will initially think that starvation is at hand. The reason that fasting works better than simply trimming down on calories is the reaction of the body at the cellular level. If you gradually reduce calories, you might actually see an increase in the build-up of fatty tissue. The body panics and responds by stocking away the food as fat tissue.

The stress response to no food is that the need for fuel will outweigh being conservative with the fat reserves. Autophagy will begin the process of eating the fat cells for energy. Your body quickly learns that there is a ready source of available energy through the fat tissue. You will begin to lose all that extra weight you've struggled with through diet after diet.

Initiating the Feast or Famine Response:

Humans have struggled with feast and famine battles throughout the ages. Empires and dynasties have been built, and many have fallen in a day. Natural disasters, fires, disease, and theft have left regions without food and famine begins. The body has learned to account for times of starvation by building up fat reserves when times are plentiful.

A complete fast is what triggers the autophagy response strongly. The body will readily dig into the reserve supplies of fat, and you will feel plenty of energy to get things done. Once you have become accustomed to fasting, you will rarely feel hungry during the process. Understanding how autophagy is keeping you fueled helps keep you motivated towards your goal. When properly prepared for a fast, you will end up feeling fully cleansed and energized.

Water Fasting and Autophagy

Water fasting is a method of deep, cellular-level cleansing that offers real results of improved health and metabolism. It's proven to be beneficial to those that are looking to maintain a good immune system, avoid degenerative illnesses and diseases, or completely sweep toxins out of the body. It can be done in inter-mittent steps or for extended amounts of time. With each round of fasting, autophagy works to clean up the cells and spaces between. Any defective or non-useful materials are cleared out, leaving a healthier environment for your cells to operate.

The Fine Art of Going Calorie-less:

Few people take the time to eat three meals a day unless one meal is through a drive-thru window. The diet in modern times is almost criminal when it comes to the nutritional needs of the human body. Most of the fast food out there are high calorie, high fat, high carb, and everything else bad for you. Shaking the habit of always having food within arm's reach has to go before starting a fast.

You can begin preparations for fasting by skipping out on a meal or two. How does it feel? Is your stomach growling and carrying on? Does it feel like you're going to starve to death? As much as it feels like it at the moment, it takes more than missing a couple of meals to starve to death. You should try and get rid of a few snack foods before starting any type of water fast. You could grab one and eat in a moment of weakness, blowing all the progress you made.

The Complete Cellular Cleanse and Detox:

All of the chemical concoctions in the world won't do the intense, deep cleaning and detox of autophagy. It can happen in a short period of time. You will reduce your chances of getting sick with viruses, bacteria, and other types of pathogens. It can even alleviate symptoms of inflammation and swelling that seem to happen for no particular reason.

When the pathways around cells and the cells themselves get hemmed up with cellular "trash" your health suffers. Cleaning everything up will ensure your cells have the best possible chance of maintaining full health and vibrance. Your metabolism will pick up, and you'll feel more energetic post-fast. It's a pain-free way to drop a few extra pounds and detox at the same time.

How Often Should You Trigger Autophagy?

Using a fasting method to trigger autophagy is fine when used sensibly. Like anything, going overboard can be more harmful than helpful. The bottom line to remember is that the fast is causing stress to your body and you will need to stop for periods and eat food. It's not recommended that you continuously fast with only tiny breaks. Be safe and check to see how you're feeling. You may have to end a fast early if it isn't feeling right. Be sensitive to the signs your body gives.

Limits on Fasting:

Intermittent water fasting is a way of depriving yourself of foods for specified periods of time that can become a lifestyle. It offers enough breaks between stages that you can find the right one for you and maintain it forever if you wish. It may even seem natural if you are a person that tends to skip a meal or two already due to being too busy to stop and eat. Missing lunch and dinner is no big deal. Extended fasting is not the same.

Extended fasting is the complete deletion of calories for 24 to 72-hours straight. All your body takes in is water. It's never recommended to water fast for more than 72-hours without the complete supervision of a doctor. It can result in health problems that can be life-threatening. The great thing is that your autophagy will be in full swing and you won't NEED to do it longer than 72-hours at a time.

Plan for Better Results:

No matter how well-suited you feel to the water fasting regime, always plan your fasts ahead of time to avoid complications that can derail the process. Choosing times that bump up against stressful holidays or bring you to gatherings with food served are the WRONG times to begin a water fast. Anyone new to fasting will find it hard to resist strong temptation with holiday meals and desserts. The same is true of family or company cook-outs, birthday parties, or business luncheons.

DO pick times that are relatively calm and look to be stress-free for the moment. The fast is already providing stress to your body. Outside stressors will only lead to frustration. Let everyone around you know that you'll be fasting so they will not bring food around, making it difficult for you to continue. You would both feel terrible if it was the temptation that made you break your fast.

DO NOT immediately get back into a fast if you had to exit one. Your body needs time to heal and recover. You also need to investigate why you broke the fast. An extended fast is tough and can come with complications. Never jump back in without knowing why it went wrong the first time.

4

THE AUTOPHAGY TIMELINE

HOW LONG DOES IT TAKE TO START SEEING RESULTS FROM autophagy? Boosting autophagy through water fasting is something that will yield great results, but you have to follow the strict plan to the end. The time frame for intermittent and extended water fasting is different, but both will give you the detox and weight loss you need. It's up to you to pick the plan that works best with your lifestyle and need for immediate results.

How Long it Takes to Initiate Autophagy

Autophagy is a natural cleaning process that is going on behind the scenes every day within your body. Fasting is a way to increase the autophagy capabilities by putting stress on the cells through food deprivation. The time table for the initiation of intense autophagy and getting results moves fast. It doesn't take months or years to see the positive benefits. All it takes is the commitment to get started.

Getting Immediate Results:

Stirring up and deepening autophagy in your body through fasting will provide almost immediate results. The key is to stay on track and avoid cheating by eating anything with calories. Fasting is used for many reasons beyond losing a few pounds of belly fat. It's the perfect detox method that's assisted through the hard work of autophagy.

Immediately after ending your fast, the resulting feeling of being free of toxins is priceless. An extended water fast will provide the biggest results, but intermittent water fasting can be done on a more routine basis. Both have their benefits and drawbacks. It should be initiated in a way that best serves your individual needs. Either can be planned for successful completion.

What to Expect:

You can fully expect to begin dropping 1 or 2 pounds of fat each week while fasting. It depends on the duration of your fast and whether you are working the intermittent or extended water fast. The more stored fat you have, the more obvious any side effects will be. Your body stores up both good and bad elements within the fat cells of your body. The results could be nausea as your body burns through these stored reserves of fuel.

Feeling a little weak or lightheaded is not abnormal until you adjust to your fast. Continued or worsening symptoms might be a reason to pause or discontinue for the time being. You can always begin your preparation process and start all over from scratch. Properly ending the fast is important. Doing this step wrong can create health problems that require medical intervention. The process of preparation will be discussed in a later chapter.

Muscle and Fat Burning:

When you first kick-start autophagy into high-gear it will allow both muscle and fat deposits to be burned as fuel. Unfortunately, this includes the heart. At some point, it will recognize that this is harmful, and autophagy will shift towards burning the fat reserves. Unlike diets that trim calories down, the body will not continue eating valuable tissues and cells during a fast.

The stress it can place on the heart is one reason it's not recommended to do an extended fast for more than 72-hours at a time. Autophagy post-fast will help repair and replace the cells that were lost, with the exception of the fat reserves. You can sabotage your results by returning to old, bad eating habits, however.

Protecting Your Heart:

It's critical to protect your heart when doing a fast. You begin this by ensuring you stay well-hydrated without drinking too much water. Water can begin to build up around the heart if you don't achieve the right balance for you. A good guideline to go by is following the same hydrating amounts of liquids you drink while not on a fast. The exception will be that all you drink is water during the fast.

Add an electrolyte water to drink during the fast. The fast can begin stripping important nutrients or water them down with a pure water diet. The electrolytes will help protect the heart and the ingredients needed to keep it beating right. Bring the fast to a safe end if you begin experiencing any heart issues.

Maximum Benefit Timeline of Autophagy

The human body is not designed to be without food for excessive amounts of time any more than it's designed to take in large amounts of food all the time. Both are extremes that can be hazardous. No matter what type of fasting you choose, they all have a window of benefit maximum before the downhill slide begins. Autophagy begins as soon as the glycogens in the liver are gone. It's usually peaking at roughly 14-16-hours into your fast. The levels of autophagy will begin to drop back down after 48-hours.

Intermittent Water Fasting:

Intermittent water fasting is the easiest of the two fasts to do, although it's not a cake walk. An intermittent fast never extends beyond an 18-hour period at the longest. It gives you a 6-hour window to fit one meal into your day and fast for the remainder.

The autophagy process begins as soon as you finish your last meal and start the water fast. The weight loss and benefits are much slower than with an extended water fast, but they are remarkable and frequent. If you practice intermittent water fasting twice a week, you can expect a loss of 1-2 pounds of fat tissue per week.

One terrific benefit of intermittent water fasting is the ability to count missed meals as fasting, which easily blends with your normal schedule. It's the type of fasting that works for busy people with tough schedules to maintain. If you eat breakfast, it might not be hard for you to skip lunch and eat a good dinner. It gives you a great deal of flexibility in choosing how much, when, and what you'll eat.

Extended Water Fasting:

Extended water fasting is a step beyond intermittent. You do not eat any food for extended hours at a time, and all you drink is water. The safe recommended period for extended fasting is 24-72 hours. Anything beyond this should be done with the helpful supervision of medical experts. The longer the fast is, the riskier it can become. You can initiate strong autophagy within the 72-hour window, so going beyond this is not necessary.

You will see the most dramatic weight loss with extended fasting within the first day or two. You will lose pounds, BUT remember it is mostly water you're losing. It will then lead to a drop in 2-4 pounds of actual body fat for a 72-hour fast. Many people opt to do a quick 24-hour extended water fast twice each week. It powers up the cleanse and detox power and promotes quick weight loss. It's easier to tackle a 24-hour water fast than the 72-hour version. It's not recommended to do a 72-hour water fast more than twice in a month. Give your body time to build nutrition and rehydrate between.

Crossing the Line:

Following the structure of the intermittent and extended water fasting routine is essential. You should never veer off and try adding time or attempt a dry fast. Dry fasting for 2-days or longer can be fatal. Every human being needs water, daily. Never ignore illness or symptoms. Your body is telling you something and you need to listen. Follow the safe stop steps in the last chapter to end the fast. Fasting can be a safe way to lose weight and detox your body, but you have to stay aware of how you're feeling during the process.

When to End the Autophagy Cycle

Ending your chosen autophagy cycle, or water fast, will depend on several factors. Riding it out to the end is preferable, but there are times it's justified to stop early. A little dizziness and weakness are to be expected if it's your first fast or you are doing an intense, extended water fast. Avoid driving or using heavy machinery during this type of fast. Keep safety in mind for you and those around you.

Sudden Illness:

Nausea is a common symptom of fasting, especially with the extended fasting. Your body has stored up all kinds of things in your fat cells. Some are toxins that will have to hit your blood-stream as they are sent out of your body via the bloodstream. Discontinue the fast if you become suddenly ill. It could be you've been invaded by a virus or bacteria while your immune system is in a weakened state.

Fasting does help the immune system in the larger picture, but at the time of fasting you are allowing your immunity defenses to go down for a brief period. Avoid fasting if anyone in your household is sick with colds, flu, viruses, or bacterial infections.

Any Heart or Kidney Problems:

Water fasting is not a safe activity for anyone that has been diagnosed with heart or liver problems. You should also discontinue a fast if you begin to feel chest pains, erratic heartbeats or a racing heartbeat. Burning urination, dark urine, or kidney pains should all signal an early exit from the fast. It could be signs of a bacterial infection or that you are not hydrated enough. The stripping of nutrients that can begin to interfere with heart activity if you are out of balance on nutrition at the start. Monitor your situation closely to avoid having to seek emergency medical treatment.

Lack of Motivation:

Everyone that fasts will hit a wall at some point during the process. A lack of motivation or a negative attitude can bring your fast to a close naturally. Try and work through the negativity and salvage the fast. Revisit all of the reasons you began a fast. Try picking your mood up and push through the low motivation. Without the right motivation you might slip and eat during the periods designed for food deprivation. Every temptation seems to take superhuman efforts to get around. If it just isn't working, end the fast safely.

You've Exceeded 72 Hours of Extended Fast:

You've battled through the 72 hours successfully. Now what? You feel a sudden urge to keep going, but do not proceed. The risks of health issues grow exponentially the longer you go past the safer 72-hour window. Congratulate yourself for making it through 72 hours but exit the fast. You can wait a week and do it all over again. The risks outweigh any benefits of continuing. As long as you eat a healthy diet, you will retain the benefits and be able to build on them with the next extended fast. It's over time that autophagy works best in both cleansing and improving your health.

You Meet Your Weight-Loss Goals:

If you started an extended or intermittent fast to lose weight, discontinue once you have reached your weight loss goal for this fasting cycle. Keep in mind that some of the weight loss will be water. It will come back once the fast is over and you begin rehydrating.

Staying too long on a fast can cause serious dehydration. Humans obtain some of the water through the foods eaten. Going back to a standard diet will bring the water weight back, but you'll be able to keep the fat burned for fuel off permanently.

Two things to monitor when using the autophagy of water fasting to lose weight are your weight and body mass index. The BMI number tells you how much body fat you have and measurements of this will show whether you are losing body fat during fasting. Set reasonable goals for each fast and end it when you get the job done. Begin planning your next fast and decide about your new weight loss goals. Each fast will continue to build on positive results.

The next chapter is important in understanding who should and shouldn't water fast. Analyze the information carefully to ensure you are in a category that will not be prone to problems with fasting. Take all the time you need to prepare and plan for your fast properly.

5

WHO SHOULD AND SHOULDN'T WATER FAST?

HOPEFULLY, YOU ARE GETTING EXCITED ABOUT ALL THE POSSIBILITIES autophagy offers you to improve health, drop weight, and increase metabolism. Before starting your first water fast you need to determine if it's safe for you to do so. Some medical conditions and other risk factors can make water fasting an impossible activity for you to try. You'll have to try another, safer method to increase autophagy in your body.

Who Will Benefit Most from Autophagy?

Everyone can benefit from a boost in the autophagy process in the body. Unless you are on the list of those that shouldn't water fast, it's a viable option you should try right away. The health benefits can be long-lasting when maintaining a healthy diet afterward.

50-Pounds and More Overweight:

Anyone that is 50-pounds and more overweight and have tried diet after diet with no success. Water fasting autophagy is a way to permanently lose weight using a natural cleansing process of the body. As long as you are in relatively good health, autophagy through fasting will help you drop the extra pounds.

Anyone Wanting a Natural Detox:

Are you tired of taking chemical potions to try and cleanse toxins and impurities out of your body? Autophagy is the most natural way to cleanse the body down to the cellular level. Detox products you buy can't do as deep of a cleansing as autophagy. You can do it several times a year without feeling any harsh side effects.

Mild to Medium Neurological Problems:

Individuals experiencing problems with memory and other cognitive functions, beginning stages of dementia, Parkinson's or Alzheimer's Disease can benefit from intermittent and extended water fasting. Make sure that the person is young enough and healthy enough to withstand the rigors of fasting.

Slow Metabolism:

Water fasting is right for every person that's felt frustrated at the slow metabolism of the body. Autophagy will give an instant boost to your metabolism that begins eating up the stored fat cells to use as energy. It doesn't require exercise, although exercise can help with the bigger picture of switching to a healthier lifestyle.

Lack of Energy:

Are you always feeling tired, even after a full night of sleep? A deep cellular cleansing might be the thing you need to feel increased levels of energy and ready to tackle the day. Both intermittent and extended water fasting will get your metabolism working more efficiently for more consistency.

Who Should Abstain from Water Fasting?

Water fasting is not the right program for everyone. The list below is not all-inclusive, and you should consult with your doctor before drastically changing your diet and eating habits. It's important that you start from a reasonably healthy point to avoid problems and discomfort.

DISCLAIMER

This book is not written by a physician and is not intended to be viewed or taken as medical advice. As with any dietary change, you should consult with your doctor to learn more about any risks associated with your particular medical situation and health condition. All information contained within this book has been thoroughly researched and is derived from sources that ARE medical experts, but it does not replace the value your personal physician's advice is to you.

Children:

Children should never be put on any type of fasting diet unless directed by and monitored through a physician. Brief fasting is sometimes required for certain blood tests or medical procedures. These are normally only an overnight fast. Growing children need a healthy amount of nutritious foods every day for their developing bodies and minds to grow optimally. Limiting sugars and watching the daily carb amounts is fine if a child is overweight, but it should be replaced with healthy foods and snacks, rather than eliminated.

Elderly:

As a person ages, the metabolism slows down and the nutrients needed to stay healthy during fasting are lost. Most elderly individuals would struggle to maintain water fasting and it could cause pre-existing medical conditions to worsen. The stress placed on every cell of the body is not recommended for someone in advanced years. The possibility of any health benefits is overridden by the risks.

Diagnosed Eating Disorders:

Anyone with an eating disorder might not be in a good place nutritionally to do fasting of any type. It can also become a new way to deprive themselves of food, creating an additional problem in their relationship with food. Fasting can simply mask an attempt at anorexic behaviors. It's better for anyone that has suffered an eating disorder to find an alternative way to increase autophagy.

Chronic Illnesses:

People suffering from chronic illnesses like leukemia, arthritis, fibromyalgia, Crohn's disease and more are not good candidates for water fasting. Many types of chronic illnesses require a variety of medications that could be troublesome during a fast. It's best to check with your doctor before embarking on a water fast.

Malnourished:

Being underweight could be an indicator that you have some level of malnourishment. Fasting does strip away nutrients from the body, and it can become a health problem if you are already lacking. Check with your doctor and see if water fasting is the best route for you to take.

Dehydrated:

Starting a water fast when dehydrated could result in kidney problems or having to drop out sooner than expected. Even though you are drinking water during the fast, you are losing all of the liquid content you get from foods. It can equate to further dehydration. Get well hydrated before starting a fast.

Heart and Kidney Problems:

The stress on tissues and organs that water fasting brings makes it risky for those with chronic kidney disease or heart problems to participate. It can cause conditions to worsen or lead to a serious medical emergency. The risk level is not worth taking. Discuss alternative cleansing or weight loss methods with your doctor.

Pregnant/Breastfeeding:

Women that are pregnant or breastfeeding need to have all available nutrients at their disposal for feeding the baby. Fasting can cause serious complications or disrupt the growth of the child. Women should wait until after breastfeeding is done.

Gout:

Gout is a type of arthritis caused by the buildup of uric acid in the body. It settles in the joints and brings on intense pain, redness, swelling, heat, and the inability to use the affected area. Water fasting can elevate uric acid in the bloodstream.

Diabetes or Hypoglycemia:

Water fasting can impact the level of blood sugar in ways that endanger someone with diabetes or hypoglycemia. The medicines used to control these conditions cannot be taken without eating or getting regular nutrition. Make attempts to adjust the blood sugar first, and your doctor might approve of water fasting further on down the line.

Prescription Medications:

Consult your doctor or pharmacist before fasting if you take any type of prescription medication. Some will not correctly absorb if you are without food. Others can cause major digestive or stomach problems when taken without food. It's better to find out than end up with problems that require medical care.

What are the Risks of Water Fasting?

As with any dietary change in eating habits, water fasting does come with some risks. It's essential to be self-aware of how you are feeling and responding during every phase of a fast. Adequate time to mentally and physically prepare are also important components of your fasting success. Most of the symptoms you feel will be at the beginning portion and should ease off as you continue with the fast. If any symptoms worsen, you might have to make a choice to pull the plug and try again another time.

Dizziness or Feeling Lightheaded:

Dizziness and lightheaded feelings during fasting are not unusual since your blood sugar levels will initially fall. Once autophagy kicks into high-gear, the dizziness should subside. Extended water fasting can result in feeling nauseated and dizzy the entire time. It's due to the toxins being removed from the body through the bloodstream.

Avoid driving or doing strenuous activities during an extended fast. You should adjust well enough to an intermittent fast that you can resume normal activities. Try drinking an electrolyte water and see if it helps balance out the situation. Don't get up from a seated position too quickly while fasting.

Muscle Weakness:

Feeling a temporary muscle weakness is not unusual when you first begin your fast. It can continue with long-lasting, extended fasts. You need to plan ahead and avoid activities that require strength and endurance during these moments. It should adjust during intermittent fasting, but an extended water fast is not the best time to enter a marathon or clean out the garage. Be careful not to do too many strenuous activities when in an extended fast. Autophagy will begin breaking down muscle tissue as well as fat, which includes the heart. It doesn't differentiate between muscles.

Extreme Deprivation of Nutrients:

Your heart depends on nutrients like potassium and magnesium to operate effectively. Long-term fasting can begin to drain you of essential elements, with no real way to bring the levels up again until you eat. It can lead to heart problems and misfiring. The stress on the heart can prove too much. You can add vitamin supplements, but they might cause stomach discomfort without food present. Begin making plans to exit the fast if you begin experiencing any problems with the heart. Don't wait for something bad to happen first. Never blow off a potential problem or think it's not serious.

Nausea and Sudden Onset Illness:

It's a guarantee that you'll feel some level of nausea when beginning your first extended water fast. The fat reserves being used as fuel are filled with all kinds of toxic materials. Nausea may come and go or disappear after a day. You may end up experiencing nausea for the duration of the fast.

Try and schedule fasts on days you don't have to work or get around town. Keep reminding yourself that it will pass once the toxins are gone. It can prove tough to push through, but you can do it. Spend more time at home if nausea is bothering you and refuses to let up.

Overhydrating:

Water fasting means you are maintaining the same amount of water in your diet as previously enjoyed, but all caloric items are gone. You need to drink the equivalent amount of water that you would without fasting. Increasing water consumption can flood out your circulatory system and create a nutrient imbalance. Drink at least 2 bottles of electrolyte water every day you are doing an extended fast. It can keep you from feeling the impact of a rush of fluids and no food. Too much water can begin building fluid up around your heart, and you'll undergo congestive heart failure.

Is Autophagy Dangerous?

The autophagy process is not harmful to the body unless you are attempting to restrict calories too much over a long period of time. Water fasting does have a dangerous side that needs to be considered in an effort to NOT fall into the actions that prove harmful.

Things to DO When Water Fasting:

- Make sure you are healthy before starting.
- Eat healthy foods and hydrate well before starting.
- Determine your normal water intake and drink the same amount.
- Discontinue fast if something doesn't feel right.
- Discontinue fast if you have symptoms of dehydration.
- Safely exit your fast.

Things to NOT DO When Water Fasting:

- Ignore warning signs from your body.
- Attempt a long fast as your first fast.
- Drink too much water.
- Continue to fast while ill.
- Fast for an unsafe length of time.
- Fast if you are on the high-risk list.

Water fasting can be a safe way to boost natural autophagy in your body and get a deeper cleanse and improved cellular actions. Good preparation and self-monitoring are key elements to fasting success. Practice is another task that will help you better prepare for how you will feel and respond to an actual water fast.

Begin fasting by attempting the intermittent water fast. Learn and master this one before heading off to the extended water fast. The next chapter will introduce you to the similarities and differences between the two. You'll have a better idea of the task ahead in entering your first fast.

6

DIFFERENCES IN INTERMITTENT AND EXTENDED WATER FASTING

Are you lost when it comes to deciding which water fasting method you need to try? This chapter will examine the highlights of each and give you the bottom line benefits for typical situations and fasting results needs. It's important to remember that both offer excellent health benefits. The difference will be the amount of time you have to devote to a fast.

Take your time and sort through your bucket list of wants to determine which one is best for you. Better planning will help you feel like you're ready. Mental preparedness is half the battle. The more informed you are about what each type of fasting consists of and how it works, the more informed your decision will be.

Choosing the Right Water Fasting Method

Your choice in water fasting methods will depend on many factors that surround your need to fast. Some people want to tap into the anti-aging and cleansing fasting provides. Others want to boost their weight loss potential. No matter what your ultimate goals are, there is a water fast that will help you meet your goal.

Sit down with a pen and paper and begin to list all the positive reasons you can think of to do a water fast. It will serve as direction to find the right one and as motivation when you are struggling to reach the goal.

Age and Health:

An extended water fast is physically demanding and mentally grueling at times. You may want to consider sticking with an intermittent water fast if you are not as spry as a 20-year-old and you live a relatively sedentary lifestyle. You could have lurking health issues you aren't aware of that an extended fast can make worse.

If you have type-2 diabetes, check with your doctor about the ability to do an extended fast. It may not be possible if you have to have medication, but you can do an intermittent fast easily.

Available Time/Schedule:

How much time do you have that can be devoted to fasting? A shorter intermittent water fast can fit into nearly any schedule, but an extended fast of 2 to 4 days will take some downtime. You will lose energy within the first two days and will have to recuperate or refeed for the same amount of time that you fast.

You can easily do a 48-hour fast if you begin on Thursday evening and end on Saturday evening. It gives you all day Sunday to eat a liquid diet and move on to soft foods by Monday. A longer fast will require dedicated time off from anything strenuous or stressful.

Fasting Goals:

What are the reasons behind fasting? Are you looking for a quicker way to lose a few pounds? Are you wanting to improve your health using the benefits of autophagy? Is a cellular-level cleansing your goal? All of these are possible using either intermittent or extended water fasting. An extended water fast will get you results faster, but multiple-day fasting can't be done as often as intermittent. It is harder to get through the longer you go. Extended fasting is perfect for those that are wanting to do an annual or semi-annual deep cleaning of the body.

Difficulty of Completing the Fast

If your schedule is normally pretty hectic and crazy, the extended water fast might not work for you. Constant interruptions or demands on your time in the middle of a deep cleansing fast can cause extreme stress and frustration. Try and time an extended fast to coincide with relaxing vacation time. Turn off your phone and enjoy the views from your window as your body works hard to remove the years of built-up toxins.

Choose a version of intermittent water fasting if you know the distractions will be completely non-stop. You can fast up to 18 hours, which about half of it can be at night as you sleep. The benefits of autophagy will be there, and you can create a regular routine to build-up the positive results.

Longer Fasts Require Deeper Commitment:

The longer you are without any calories and dining on pure water, the deeper your commitment will have to be towards the fast. Temptations will come along and try to derail your progress. The best planning in the world can't keep the mind from wandering to thoughts of food during the first couple of days of an extended water fast.

The battle is not just a physical one in which your body wants food. It's a mental hurdle to overcome the intense feelings of hunger and ignore the tummy growling. It DOES get easier as it goes along, but initially, it's rough. If you can ride out the first 36 hours, the other 12 hours on a 48-hour fast go by quickly.

Temporary Loss of Energy:

If you choose to do a 48 to 72-hour extended water fast, you will feel an energy drain between days 2 and 3. Your body is using much of the energy it generates to root out and get rid of toxins in your body. Your autophagy is in full performance mode. Stay away from doing any sort of strenuous physical activity due to the lack of energy, possible dizziness, and autophagy that can begin to dine on your muscle tissues when exerted.

An intermittent water fast is not as draining on your energy levels. You will have enjoyed a meal sometime within the past 24-hours. The deprivation is not as deep but still yields good results.

Difficulty with Symptoms:

The symptoms that can accompany a fast when you are ill-prepared can be difficult. You should stay in tune with how your body is feeling, your emotional state, and whether anything feels "off." The symptoms of an extended fast can become seriously troubling in a hurry. If you become disoriented at any point or ill, get medical attention right away.

The great thing about fasting is that if you begin to be bothered by intense hunger pains, end the fast. The solution is that simple. End it the right way, however. Don't just run out and grab a cheeseburger. Drink pure liquids the first day and soft foods the next. Anything more than this can cause you to get sick or seriously mess with your blood sugar levels.

Which Fast is More Effective?

The effectiveness of the fast you choose is relative to the results you need. Both intermittent and extended water fasting are incredibly effective in different ways. Intermittent is better for frequent, long-term use and extended is beneficial for the occasional long fast or more frequent 24-hour fasts.

Beginning fasters should start with the intermittent fast to get a feel for what the experience is like. Using the right intermittent fast can work well as a bridge to move on into the deeper, extended fast. It can work seamlessly, requiring little thought or effort.

Deep Detoxing:

The extended water fast is the best one for performing deep cleansing and detox. The ability to focus the autophagy on cleaning details in and around your cells for up to 72 hours will provide the deepest natural cleanse possible, safely. You should never run a longer water fast without being supervised by medical personnel. If you run into problems, having medical experts handy can help you get the medical treatment you need.

An 18-hour intermittent water fast can also offer some deep cleansing results, but not to the level of a fast that goes for days. Frequent cycling of longer intermittent fasting can get deeper results, but they are only seen over time. Extended water fasting provides more immediate results.

Permanent Weight Loss:

Both types of water fasting offer permanent weight loss benefits. The results are equivalent to the time spent fasting. The extended fast can last up to 4 days, with a normal initial loss of 3 pounds in water and an additional 1 or 2 pounds per day of stored fat. It equates to an amount of up to 11 pounds for the extended fast. A 1-hour intermittent water fast will yield the same 3 pounds of water loss and about 1 pound of body fat.

A longer extended water fast is perfect if you want to drop that last stubborn 3 or 4 pounds to fit into your wedding dress. Use the steady weight loss potential offered by intermittent water fasting for continued weight loss.

Extensive Autophagy:

Autophagy will be running at full throttle by your 12th hour of fasting, no matter which method you use. The methods are equal in an ability to sort through and begin removing harmful things from your system. How you at the end will be similar in increased energy, less fatigue, faster metabolism, and a sense of well-being.

If you are wanting to try autophagy to detox and remove bad cells from your body, or try to inhibit the growth of tumors, the longer extended water fast is better. It can take up to 7-days for autophagy to begin disposing of tumor growth, but the 72-hour window allows your body to begin inhibiting the growth. Specific extended water fasting to try and beat cancer should only be done under the care of a doctor.

Will the Fasting Results Last?

Lasting results are what every person wants when they put in as much effort and time as the preparation and completion that serious fasting requires. Will your expected results happen? If so, will they last? The answer to both can be yes if you aren't looking for pie-in-the-sky results from one fast and are willing to maintain healthy eating habits after the work is done.

Fat and Water Losses:

Prepare to feel disappointment if you are a scale hopper! The first couple of pounds, at least, are pure water loss from not eating foods during the fast. You will immediately regain this once you are off the fast. It can be disappointing to see that your total weight loss is only 2 pounds, depending on the type and length of fast.

Knowing this piece of information ahead of time will help you come to terms with the fact that weight loss is not the only benefit of autophagy. The removal of toxins from your system that have built up over time has far-reaching health benefits. You have the ability to reduce your odds of getting diseases or neurodegenerative conditions drastically.

Weight Maintenance for the Long-Term:

Cleaning out your body at the cellular level will increase your metabolism. It serves as a way to better maintain a healthy weight once you get there. At surface level, the results might not appear to be stunning, but the ongoing benefits will give you results that are priceless. Youthful appearance, feel, improved ability to fight disease, and improved cognitive abilities can all be had by following the intermittent or extended water fasting plans.

Consider Switching to a Ketogenic Diet:

A diet that consists of roughly 75 percent fats, 20 percent protein, and 5 percent carbs is what is referred to as a ketogenic diet. It forces the body to burn fat for energy instead of breaking down carbs to sugars. It puts you in a state of ketosis. It's essential not to overdo the proteins or use lean meats. Fatty fish or grass fed beef works well.

Going on a ketogenic diet will help provide you with backup autophagy all the time. You can continue to enjoy some of the benefits of a fast without fasting all the time. Spend two days each week using the keto diet and it will help you maintain the progress you made during the fast. The wide variety of foods you can use with keto diets makes it a popular way to switch to a healthier lifestyle.

Now it's time to learn how to begin your first fast. Are you ready? Well, keep reading!

7

HOW TO PREP FOR AND BEGIN INTERMITTENT WATER FASTING

WELCOME TO THE CHAPTER THAT WILL KICK OFF YOUR JOURNEY INTO intermittent water fasting. The amount of preparation you do should be equivalent, or equal to the time you spend doing any important activity. If you want to have a successful experience in intermittent water fasting, be willing to put in some quality time preparing.

This book will only focus on four types of intermittent water fasting even though there are many more. It's one of the most varied and flexible in all aspects of food choices, restriction methods, and duration of fasting states. In other words, there's hardly any way you can go wrong. Less complicated is good, right? Mental preparation is your reasonable first step.

How to Mentally Prepare for an Intermittent Water Fast

Your mental focus and positive framing will be as critical for your fasting success as your physical ability to stick with the program. Negativity received from others and dealing with stress from without the body can make the battle inside tougher. Spend a decent amount of time planning, strategizing, and digging for deep motivation. You'll be ready to hit the ground running if you begin the mental preparation at least two weeks prior to your fast. It's one of the best things you can do with your spare time, especially if you're serious about trying your first intermittent water fast.

Keep Focused on the Health Benefits:

Not too many activities associated with dietary changes allow you to reap the ongoing benefits of autophagy. Intermittent water fasting is one that is simple to do and can fit into the busiest of schedules. It's one of the most flexible ways to boost your health. It's a dietary change in routine that can fit the most active lifestyle. It's time to revisit the list you made earlier about all the reasons for starting a fasting routine.

When you turn your focus to all the positive aspects, you'll relax and begin to look forward to starting the day. The use of autophagy for a natural body detox is a way of looking after your health for the years to come. Most people allow toxins to build up for years, which can lead to chronic illness and disease that can cause excessive pain, inflammation, loss of mobility, or premature death. Routine cleansing will reduce the risks of toxin-induced health troubles.

Find and Read Success Stories for Motivation:

You may feel even more prepared for fasting success by finding real testimonials and stories of people just like you that tried intermittent water fasting and loved it! You can find numerous websites that are filled with the real stories of individuals that struggled to lose weight, battled potential illness, or suffered from sluggish metabolism and felt almost immediate relief after beginning a fasting routine.

Begin a blog page of your own to share your personal experiences.

You might motivate someone else to take the same journey you are about to embark on. Finding ways to connect with others that have been in your shoes can be the best way to alleviate any concerns you have about whether you can stick with it long enough to make a difference. New and unknown experiences can always make you feel a little wary, but the health benefits of intermittent water fasting are too great to walk away from without giving it an honest try.

See if there are any local groups that promote the ketogenic or fasting lifestyle. Creating friendships in this process is an even greater benefit. It gives you like-minded people to use as a support when the day is rough and you want to ditch the fast.

Avoid Negative People and Negative Emotions:

Negativity is one of the biggest killers of motivation. In preparing for starting your first intermittent water fast, avoid people that offer nothing but negative thoughts, statements, and energy. It's not worth mentioning your plans if it will only end up in a big negative debate. If you are surprised by a sudden negative opinion given about your plans, change the subject or walk away. Keep your energy and thoughts positive. It's not worth getting into an argument if the results won't affect the outcome. You'll still do your fasting and they'll still not like it.

Negative emotions are just as bad in your attempts to stay positive. Look for ways to alleviate and control stress levels pre-fast. The fasting will already be a stress to the body. Added emotional stress and negativity can hinder your ability to focus and complete the fast. You need to have a positive and calm atmosphere at least for the starting point of the fast. You might want to hold off if everything seems to be making you aggravated, upset, or frustrated. It's better to wait a week for a better time than have everything go crazy in the middle of your first fast.

Plan and Stay Organized:

Plan everything about your upcoming intermittent water fast down to the last detail. Find out more about anything you don't fully understand with the upcoming fast. The more you know, the more successful it'll be. Make the most sensible plan to start with that leads you to a successful outcome. It will motivate you to keep pushing limits. Start with the fasting plan that seems easiest to you and work up from there. You can eventually level up to try an extended fast. Get the feel of how fasting affects your body first.

Have everything you need for your fast before you start. That includes all the elements of foods you are eating pre-fast and the re-feeding products you might need. Typically, re-feeding isn't a necessary part of intermittent fasting, but you might feel more comfortable with soft or liquid foods for your first meal afterward. Whatever you think you'll need should be ready and available at the time you start. Post your plans in an area that is easy to see, such as the refrigerator door. It's another simple way to keep you motivated and looking forward to your fast.

Let Everyone in on the Plan:

Everyone that is close to you and will be interacting with you during the fast should be told about your plans. It gives you a broader base of support and can help eliminate possible temptation by those that have no idea you are fasting. No one wants to have to turn away fresh baked cookies and it can bring about a huge mental dilemma that's hard to win. Well, cookies usually win, which means your fast will be broken from the start. Avoiding this little problem is as easy as letting everyone know you are entering a fast and won't be eating for a bit.

It's also important that people aware of your fasting if you live alone. Having someone check on you and how you're doing is important for your emotional support and physical safety. It can be a neighbor, co-worker, relative, or friend.

How to Physically Prepare for an Intermittent Water Fast

Physically preparing to enter an intermittent water fast can help you gain an understanding of what you'll experience before you even start. The things you do here in the prep stage can determine your success. Take all of the necessary time you need to experiment and feel comfortable before rushing headlong into the fast.

Switch to a Low Carbohydrate Diet and Reduce Portion Sizes:

Adjusting what you eat and how much can go a long way towards preparing you for an intermittent water fast. A reduction in carbohydrates, sugars, and eliminating processed foods will get your body more receptive to the fast you enter. Change your drinking habits to non-sugar drinks like herbal teas, coffee, and plain water. Don't add sugar or creamer to your coffee or tea to avoid the extra calories.

Begin reducing the portion size of the food you serve yourself. It might seem like a little thing, but it will help to begin shrinking your stomach before the big day. The fast might seem easier if you didn't have to listen to and feel your tummy rumble for hours on end. Begin by tossing back half the protein and keep the veggies. Eliminate dessert if it's been a daily favorite. The more excess you trim from your eating now, the easier the fast will be.

Drink Plenty of Water and Discover Your Baseline:

How much water do you drink each day? How much water are you supposed to drink each day? The recommended 8 to 10 glasses is something that very few people actually do. It's closer to 4 or 6 glasses, depending on your weight and height. Spend some time figuring out what your normal baseline amount is and have the same amount set aside in bottled form. You need to know what your actual average daily intake is so that you don't over-hydrate during your fast.

Skip Breakfast One Day and Breakfast and Lunch the Next:

Discover how your body responds to a lack of food by giving it a trial run. Skip breakfast one day. Go ahead and eat a normal lunch and dinner. You may not be too affected by one skipped meal, especially since many people opt to skip breakfast anyway. It's not a bad way to start a fast. Mornings are usually one of the busiest times of day for everyone. All the rushing around to get to work and breakfast is hardly missed.

The very next day you need to skip breakfast and lunch. How are feeling by about mid-afternoon? Are you noticing any change in blood sugar levels? Is there any dizziness or feeling lightheaded? Note any major symptoms you recognize and write them down. It gives you an idea of how your body will react to real fasting.

Make sure you continue to hydrate as normal. Skipping food doesn't mean skipping your glass of water. Drink it at the normal time that would be your meal. It will help your stomach feel fuller for a few moments. Don't drink any more than normal to compensate for the lack of food. It leads to over-hydration, which can kill you. Do this process a few times before committing to the fast. You'll become a professional before you ever start.

Skip All Meals for an Entire Day:

Once you feel you have the two-meal deletion mastered, it's time to move on to skipping all meals for an entire day. It shouldn't be a huge ordeal if you've already been cutting down on your portion sizes. The evening meal is usually the biggest of the day and the one that most women miss. It's a time of social interaction and eating with family. Substitute a warm cup of herbal tea and socialize with the family anyway. You can replace it with broth if you find that your mind won't come off thoughts about food. You can wean off this after a couple of tries.

Make sure everyone in your house understands that you're preparing for a fast and not developing an eating disorder. Young adults that still live at home could have problems starting if a parent overthinks the actions or inactions of their grown child. Give the necessary reassurances and show them some information online about intermittent water fasting and the obvious health benefits. It may not keep the parent from worrying, but at least they won't be talking like you need to get emergency psychiatric help. You'll have one more person in your corner.

Eliminate Snacks at Least Two Weeks Before Fasting:

Who needs real food when there are a hundred snacks to try? Gather up all of your snack items and get them out the door. Give them to friends, family, or toss them in the trash. Leave no chips, cookies, or snack cake items that are easy to grab and a big no-no. You can switch to an alternative form of snack that is healthy, such as vegetables and low-fat ranch dressing, or saltine crackers and your favorite sliced cheese. Use the cheese sparingly since fasting can sometimes bring on constipation. You might be surprised at how much money gets spent junk.

Make it a rule to quit buying food when you're out away from your home. Fast food has been one of the biggest problems and contributors when it comes to childhood and adult obesity. Allowing a child to grow up with a poor understanding of nutrition and real nutritional needs will guarantee he/she struggles financially, educationally, and never have a mind of their own. Spend time learning about the basics of sound nutrition and where the lines need to be drawn with unhealthy food choices.

How to Begin an Intermittent Water Fast

Once you've accomplished all the preparatory work that's helpful, you can choose your plan and start the intermittent water fast. All the ones listed below are easy and rather uncomplicated in nature. You can find a thousand ways fasting plans have been changed, modified, and whittled to fit particular schedules and lifestyles. I would encourage you to check out the myriads of options available.

You can always add fruit juice at meal time if you are struggling to get through a multi-hour fast. You must be forgiving of yourself if it takes a little time and practice to become a champ. Switch to another fast if the one you try doesn't seem a good fit. Intermittent water fasting is full of options and flexible ways to customize the fasting.

Lean/Gains:

The lean gains water fast is geared towards anyone that wants to lean out their muscles and control body fat content. It works well as a way to trigger autophagy and get the deep cleanse you need. Women using this intermittent water fasting method have to stick to a daily routine of 14-hours total fast. You can drink normal amounts of water but no food intake. The remaining 10-hours can include food. A one-week schedule of this routine would look like this:

Monday: 14h-complete fast/ 10h-eat

Tuesday: 14h-complete fast/ 10h-eat

Wednesday: 14h-complete fast/ 10h-eat

Thursday: 14h-complete fast/ 10h-eat

Friday: 14h-complete fast/ 10h-eat

Saturday: 14h-complete fast/ 10h-eat

Sunday: 14h-complete fast/ 10h-eat

It's a repetitive schedule, but you can work it around to fit your workout routines or your work schedule. The only problem with this plan is that you have to be very disciplined. You have 10 hours available to eat whatever you want. Binge eating can be a problem.

It's a nice fasting program in that you don't have to go too many hours at one time. Pretty much anyone can handle this program. You can get a feel for the fasting phase and the feeding phase and how the two complement one another.

Eat – Skip – Eat:

The eat-skip-eat water fast is pretty straightforward. You choose two days of the week to completely fast and the rest you can eat as you would normally. It gives you training and discipline to make it through complete days of fasting. A sample week schedule would look like this:

Monday: Eat

Tuesday: Eat

Wednesday: Fast

Thursday: Eat

Friday: Eat

Saturday: Fast

Sunday: Eat

The days of the week chosen to eat or fast are completely up to you. It's a great fasting program that can lead you into doing the extended water fast. Once again, you need to be guarded about eating too much on the days you are unrestricted.

Warrior Diet:

Another great intermittent water fasting routine is called the Warrior diet. It's supposedly derived from our ancestral selves that would have hunted all day and ate for four hours in the cave at night or something along these lines. All you have to do is fast with water only for 20 hours, and then you can eat during the remaining 4-hour window.

Monday: 20h-fast/ 4h-eat

Tuesday: 20h-fast/ 4h-eat

Wednesday: 20h-fast/ 4h-eat

Thursday: 20h-fast/4h-eat

Friday: 20h-fast/4h-eat

Saturday: 20h-fast/ 4h-eat

Sunday: 20h-fast/ 4h-eat

It's another fasting technique that can be used to bridge over to the extended water fast by switching to the long fast instead of eating for the remaining 4-hour period. You'll already be 20 hours into the extended water fast!

Alternate Day Fasting:

The alternate day fast is more of a diet than fast, but there is a reason it's included in this book. Rather than a true fast, you are driven down to a restricted 400 to 500 caloric intake diet on the light days. The alternating days you're allowed to eat as normal. It's included because not much is required to switch this from light days to the eat-skip-eat plan. Easy methods to bridge and move forward are always appreciated. You can get used to the restricted calories first and then jump to the actual fasting program.

Monday: Light-Calorie

Tuesday: Normal

Wednesday: Light-Calorie

Thursday: Normal

Friday: Light-Calorie

Saturday: Normal

Sunday: Light-Calorie

No matter what type of intermittent fast you choose, you'll enjoy how flexible and easy they are to fit your schedule. You can continue with these types of fasts continuously if you choose. Many people build their entire lives around the fasting schedule, which means they have faith in the results. Give one a try and see how it works for you.

How to Detect Problems with the Intermittent Fast

It's wise to closely self-monitor your health as you move through your intermittent water fast. Catching problems early can keep you from ending up in the hospital. Thankfully, most problems can be corrected by ending the fast. It can seem disappointing, but it's better to look after your health enough to try the fast again at another time. Always stop the fast in a safe manner when you have symptoms that involve the heart or the kidneys.

Nausea or Vomiting When Ending Fasting Period:

Nausea and feeling a little "off in the tummy" is not at all unusual with any type of fast. You are depriving the body of nutrients and it is seeking a source internally. Shorter fasts should not offer any type of serious stomach cramp and nausea issues, but the longer 14 or 18-hour fast can be made difficult with nausea. The nausea symptoms should go away after you end the fast and take in nutrients.

Experiencing nausea and throwing up after ending the fast could indicate you are transitioning back to a "normal" diet too quickly. Your body is unable to move as fast as your mind wants it to. Back off and try a half day of nothing but fruit juice in the place of a meal. Use it as a guide for the next fast. Your body requires a little extra adjustment time.

Migraine Headache:

Have you ever had what many people term as a "hungry headache?" It can feel like someone is gouging your eyeballs out with a hot fireplace poker. Well, in reality, it is more likely due to a lack of proper hydration. Migraines are a typical sign of dehydration. You can increase the amount of water you're drinking but it may not help. It's better to end the fast and try again in a few days after hydrating more.

Look for other signs of dehydration like excessively dry skin, constant thirst, and darker urine. Readjust your level of water intake and make sure the right hydration is in place before attempting your next fast. The extra uric acid that hits your system during fasting can be complicated with dehydration. You can end up with irritated kidneys, bladder, or both.

A good indication that your renal system is in good shape for a fast is to have bright, almost clear urine and in plentiful supply. You should be completely headache-free. Wait to fast until you have the perfect window of opportunity.

Extreme Dizziness:

Fasting has a direct impact on the blood sugar level in your body. It can also lower your blood pressure. Either one of these can be responsible for causing dizziness. Small amounts of lightheaded feelings are nothing to worry about. Feeling extremely dizzy or as if you are going to pass out is something to look at closely. Is the dizziness all the time or only when you stand up and sit down? Are you experiencing any unusual or erratic heartbeats? If the dizziness goes away when at rest, it might be an indication you entered the fast too quickly or are still trying to adjust.

You need to end the fast if it's a matter of a drop in blood sugar. Those with diabetes type-2 and borderline diabetes can have blood sugar readings that are all over the map at times. Drink a glass of juice and see if the dizziness subsides. You may have to plan on fasting another day when your blood sugar is in a normal range. Stressing yourself out worrying about the fasting experience can also contribute to the problem. Try and stay in a relaxed frame of mind, fasting or no fasting.

Stomach Cramps and Intense Hunger:

The first few times you fast, even for short periods, can be tough. Your body wants nutrition that's readily available when it wants it. It can't be bothered you're trying to do something healthy. Your stomach starts demanding food. Other than being slightly embarrassing when in public and slightly uncomfortable, a little stomach cramping and rumbling won't hurt anything. Try and push through if you can. The longer you go, the less the stomach will revolt. It gets easier.

A feeling of intense hunger is different. Your body is sending you a strong signal that this might not be the time you complete a fast. Ignoring a few stomach rumblings is one thing. Ignoring the body that's telling you it's absolutely starving is not good. Chalk it up as a temporary setback and try fasting again another time. It can take a few tries before reaching success with longer intermittent water fasts. Make sure you properly ease out of the fast and don't take things too quickly. The last chapter in this book will focus on safe fasting exits.

Sudden Loss of Energy:

Most intermittent water fasting routines are so brief that you shouldn't experience much in the way of muscle weakness or sluggishness. It's possible with the 14 to 18-hour fast under the right conditions. Any fast is going to leave you with less energy than you would have if in the feeding state. You need to account for this possibility if you're planning a longer fast. Avoid strenuous activity or anything that requires detailed attention. You'll most likely want to hang out or catch a nap.

Low energy can be a sign that your blood sugar level has dropped. You can try a few sips of juice if the condition is problematic or seems serious. You might find that a small glass of juice provides enough lift that you can finish your fast. The body's sensitivity to insulin and a lack of readily available food can cause a sudden drop in blood sugar without any long-term effects.

8

HOW TO PREP FOR AND BEGIN EXTENDED WATER FASTING

Extended water fasting is a way to get the deepest natural body cleansing possible. It's not an activity for the faint of heart but the results in complete deep cellular cleansing are worth the effort. Paying close attention to how your body is responding during this type of intense fast is important. You can end up with a problem that gets out of control quickly. It's safe as long as you closely monitor and follow the safe exit plan. Knowing when to say enough with the long fast is also a great skill to develop. Let's begin by learning how to prepare for an extended fast mentally.

How to Mentally Prepare for an Extended Fast

Preparing for an extended water fast takes a few of the ideas from the intermittent fast and expands on the skills and mindset. The difference in the shorter intermittent fasting and extended are dramatic when it comes to mental fortitude and the need to push through barriers. The difference is depriving your body of nutrients for a few hours versus actual days at a time.

Understanding the Mental Battle of the Long Fast:

You will experience some of the same physical symptoms as intermittent water fasting initially, but it will gradually progress into a different world. The long extended fast that goes beyond 24 hours is one that takes mental and physical preparation in order to see it through to completion. You won't always succeed, but the autophagy benefits you receive are yours to keep.

Getting through a 72-hour extended water fast will be a feat that is likened to reaching the summit of a mountain as a climber. Each time you reach it, there's cause for celebration. There's no need to go beyond the safe zone of 72 hours since you've reached maximum autophagy benefits by day 2. As drained as you feel afterward, you know that autophagy cleared out a bunch of trash and gunk that had built up in your body for years. You can now get back to living with a clean internal slate.

Expectations of Mood Swings:

An extended water fast will have your emotions and thinking all over the map. The hormonal imbalances and fluctuating chemicals in your system will have you up one minute and down the next. It can seem like a never-ending roller coaster ride. Mood swings are an entirely natural part of the process and to be expected. It can be rough on those around you that care and don't quite understand why you're so moody. It's a good thing to have a discussion about this topic before you begin your extended fast. Everyone being on the same page is helpful.

You can pre-plan for the ups and downs by having a few creature comforts around that make you happy. Keep a good book handy to read, a good movie to watch, or a soft blanket to tuck over you and get some much-needed rest. You should treat the long fast as a time of rest and repair. It might be a good time to connect with any people you have located in your community that are also extended water fast believers. As the days move on you will have less energy to do things and will primarily sleep.

When Your Body Betrays Your Spirit:

As much as you want to make it all the way through this fast, your body may betray you and cause the end of the fast early. Your first instinct is to feel crushing disappointment but is it really a failure? The level of commitment and focus on details to get yourself to this point should not be lost in the disappointment of having to end the fast. It's to be expected that not every fast attempt will work out due to a mix of conditions that are not fully met. The times you are able to complete a full 72-hour fast are to be savored.

Are you really ready to call the fast or do you just need a quick infusion of nutrition? A dose of electrolyte water or a small cup of juice can't hurt. It might give you the balance and strength to make it the last few yards. You don't really lose anything by having to end a fast for comfort or safety reasons. You've still gained some great detox deep down to your cellular components. It's one time you will walk away a winner, no matter the outcome.

Dealing with Zero Energy Levels:

A few safety concerns will come up when planning for your extended water fast. You should feel wonderful the first day, extremely hungry the second day and then a big wall of exhaustion should hit. It seems to take real effort to do anything, including think. Your body is now in complete ketosis and is feeding off the fat stores. The energy derived seems different and like a foreign currency. Your body is not quite sure how or where to spend the money. The thought process you relied upon to get you to this point seems to be taking a hit as well. Everything is in slow-motion.

No matter how independent you are as a person, you need to have someone near that can check on you frequently and help motivate you when the exhaustion wall hits. If your bedroom is upstairs, get help going up and down the stairs to avoid falling. If you do need emergency services, someone should be there to make the call and monitor your condition.

When Should I Say, "I'm Done?"

The decision to pull the plug will largely be your decision, but you should follow the advice of others around you that might see things a bit clearer. If they feel you've done enough then just call the end to the fast. It's not worth jeopardizing your health to make some personal record of fasting. If all you make it through is 48 hours, you have 48 hours-worth of hardcore autophagy in your favor.

You can feel confident that anytime you are feeling uncomfortable or that it's too much, it's okay to stop the fast. Follow the safe exit procedure in the last chapter to avoid any health problems as you leave the fast and begin the re-feed process. It can become a life-threatening situation if you try to jump on regular foods too fast after a long water fast.

How to Physically Prepare for an Extended Fast

A few more physical preparations are in order for an extended water fast than for the intermittent variety. You need to prepare for the large energy drain you'll feel after day 2, although some can experience it earlier. It's not recommended that you do a full 72-hour extended water fast without attempting a few at lesser amounts of time. It helps to see how your body reacts to the stress of complete food deprivation for days on end. Although each person reacts individually, there are some basics that remain the same no matter who is fasting.

Good Nutrition and Hydration:

Eating good nutritious foods, especially in the days before your extended fast, is important for having the right building blocks to set as your foundation. Proper hydration is necessary before, during, and after the fast. Try to avoid drinking excessive amounts of water. Spread it out over the time of your fast. Water is not designed to replace the food. You can end up with a dangerous imbalance of electrolytes by drinking too much water.

Following the keto diet or drastically reducing your carbs will be beneficial in the days or weeks before starting the extended water fast. A reduction in the number of meals and meal portions will also be helpful in preparing for days of no meals. Eat a well-balanced diet when it comes to essential nutrients.

Practice Using Intermittent Fasting:

Intermittent water fasting can be your inspiration and launching pad for preparing to tackle the more rigorous extended water fast. Everything you need to do in order to prepare for the intermittent fast is beneficial to the extended fasting. It makes sense that you would utilize the tools of one to prepare for the other. The intermittent fasting will demonstrate the complete feeling of living without eating meals. The transition to an extended diet should be smoother with a few intermittent water fasting sessions under your belt.

Take good notes during an intermittent water fast about how you are feeling and how your body is responding. Write down any areas you struggled to get through. What were some things you found helpful? What were some things you found hindering progress? It's invaluable information if you can set it to help firm up your planning for the extended fasting. In the meantime, every bit of fasting you do is allowing autophagy to clean out your body and improve your health. It's a complete win-win solution.

Have Someone in Place to Check in on You:

Entering an extended water fast is not a time to become fiercely independent. You need to plan ahead and have a dependable person available to stay with you or frequently check on you while you fast and recover. You will end up in a weakened state near the end of a long fast and can get hurt by falling or experience a medical emergency. What would happen if you needed to call someone, but the phone slipped off the bed and you didn't have the energy to retrieve it? It's always better to be safe and have help at your access.

Having someone around also helps break the monotony of not being able to get around much. You at least have someone to talk to when you're bored and don't have the energy to read or stay focused on a movie plot. It's also someone you can discuss with about any symptoms you have that are worrisome to you. It can help to have a sounding board to determine when you should end a long fast. The other person may notice problems that you aren't seeing. Make sure you involve someone you trust so that you can allow their opinions and voice to hold merit in your decision-making process.

Make Sure Nothing Strenuous Needs Done During Your Fast:

After starting an extended fast is NOT the time to give your dog a bath, do the grocery shopping, vacuum the downstairs, and do a ton of laundry. You need to prepare to do less and less as time marches on. Your energy will be dwindling, and you might feel fairly unsteady on your feet at times. It helps if you aren't the only one in the household. You can always defer daily chores to the other people while you fast. Some of the larger tasks should be done before the fast or after you finish the re-feeding.

The two main reasons to avoid strenuous activity are the fact that in a weakened state you can fall or trip and get hurt. The second is that you will have tremendous autophagy happening which can begin eating away at muscles when active. At this point, the fast would be working against you. Plan, prepare, and plan again to have everything done you need before beginning your fast. The actual fasting period should be treated more like a complete luxurious relaxation. Push off stress and enjoy this time of complete and deep healing for your body.

Using Intermittent Fasting as a Bridge:

Not only can the intermittent water fasting work as a practice run at the extended version, but you can actually use it as a bridge to begin your longer fast. You can time a longer intermittent fast to end in the morning hours and simply continue on as an extended fast. You will have already made it through one day with little to no effort. Follow all the prep advice for starting the intermittent fast and you'll be fine to continue on with the extended version. It's another reason why you should do a few trial runs with the intermittent fast and get used to the routine.

Jumping into an extended fast without preparation is dangerous. No matter which way you decide to go, make sure you do your prep work and monitor your health. It's better to end a fast early for health reasons than to end up in the hospital.

You now have all the information you need to begin an extended water fast. The following information will give you step-by-step instructions on how to start and what to look for when problems arise. Don't start the program until you feel you are completely ready. There's never a reason to rush.

How to Begin an Extended Water Fast

Two ways exist in which to begin your extended water fast. You can bridge it over as an extension of an intermittent water fast or try it cold turkey. The latter is more difficult if you have never fasted before and is not the preferred method, but with plenty of preparation, you can make it work. The extended water fast carries the most risk of side effects and problems. Take proper precautions and check in with yourself every so often to see how you're holding up.

Extended Water Fast Following Intermittent Water Fast:

Bridging from Warrior Diet –

The Warrior Diet is the 20-hour fast and 4-hour eat daily schedule. Bridging it is as easy as dropping the 4-hour eating portion and continue the complete fast.

Bridging from Lean/Gains –

Lean/gains is the 14-hour fast and 10-hour eat. Bridge by dropping the 10-hour eating portion and continue the complete fast.

Bridging from Eat-Skip-Eat –

The Eat-Skip-Eat is an alternating eat-fast routine. To bridge to the extended diet, switch the next eat day in line to complete fast.

As you can see above, bridging from the intermittent water fasting routines is easy and not hard to figure out how to put them together.

Extended Water Fast Without Intermittent Water Fast:

Beginning the extended water fast from scratch will take a little more time for preparation if you are not already involved in a fasting program. You should begin a routine of alternating days of eating and juice fasting. Juice fasting is replacing a meal with an 8-10-ounce glass of juice. You should do this for 2 weeks.

The next two weeks you should alternate eat-fast days. Pick a fast day at the end of your two weeks and jump right into the extended fast. The benefit is you already have one fast day down.

Pay close attention to your body and look for any symptoms that are problematic. Stop the fast if you are feeling uncomfortable or ill in any way. It's much better to be safe when it comes to your health and overall well-being.

How to Detect Problems with the Extended Water Fast

Extended water fasting is not without its share of risks and problems. All the problems listed below are valid reasons to stop the fast quickly and possibly seek immediate medical attention. It is one reason you should never attempt an extended fast without having someone close by that can help you if things go sour. Not every long fast will end abruptly but the cases below are good reasons to try it again another time.

Migraine Headaches that Worsen:

If you are sensitive to blood sugar levels and frequently get migraines from missing a meal, the extended fast might not be the right fit for you. Imagine how powerful the headaches can become after missing multiple meals? In the fasting state, you won't be able to take aspirin or other product to relieve the pain, or it will cause a stomach bleed or upset. You are either stuck in a state of misery or forced to end the fast early.

Migraine headaches can also be a signal that you are seriously dehydrated. You can try increasing the water you're drinking and see if it helps. If nothing seems to be relieving the pain, use the safe exit route and try the fast another time.

Suddenly Falling Ill:

Never, ever, ever start an extended fast if you have so much as a sniffle. That small sneeze or cough can flare up into a raging illness such as the flu or pneumonia that gets out of control quickly. The fasting state allows the body to concentrate energy on cleaning old cell parts and pieces and detox the cells of the body. The lowering of the defenses can allow a virus or bacteria to hop on in and attack. It's unsafe to continue a long fast when you're seriously ill.

Who knows what is being brought out of your body by the autophagy process? It will bring every toxin that's been stored in your body for years to your bloodstream for permanent disposal. A large number of toxins in your blood can make you ill. The best thing to do is discontinue the fast and see your doctor if the illness doesn't ease up. A little bit of nausea is common when fasting, but you should never be full-on sick. It means your body might need a slower detox that is more tolerable. You might have to backtrack and stick with the intermittent water fast.

Unusual Heart Activity:

Any problems that crop up involving the heart function or a serious drop in blood pressure are a major concern. You need to end the fast immediately and safely, and ask questions later. You may not notice a problem right away but the longer the fasting goes, the more it's stripping your body of the nutrients it needs to support heart and cardiovascular activity. The only cure for this is to restart nutrient supplies. If you do nothing it can lead to cardiac arrest. Don't play around when it has to do with the heart or circulatory system.

You might notice a periodic "fluttering" of the heart, missed beats, or a sudden racing heartbeat. You might suddenly feel dizzy. Have someone monitor your pulse and have a blood pressure monitor close by. Call an ambulance if the symptoms persist or seem to get worse. Use the gentle and easy re-feeding technique in the last chapter to reintroduce nutrients to your body. Call an ambulance if you end up having chest pains or show any signs of a heart attack. The stress on the entire body by extended fasts is not tolerable by anyone with heart problems. Please avoid fasting if you have heart disease or a limiting condition.

Bad Leg Cramps:

Leg cramps can hit out of the blue and make you feel miserable. It feels like a huge Charlie horse right at the back of your legs and all you can really do is writhe around the bed in pain. Massaging doesn't really do much until it decides to back off. What is the cramping all about? Can you believe it's as simple as having your levels of magnesium drop too low? It will begin making your legs and arms cramp and cause extensive pain. The real worry is that your heart depends on magnesium as well for the firing action. If levels of magnesium have dropped to the point that your muscles suffer, your heart is having trouble too.

Fix a small glass of juice with any fruits or vegetables that are high in magnesium. Drinking this should make the pain and cramping go away. You can go on with the fast if you want but it might be wiser to discontinue and get your vitamin and nutrient level up before another fast. You don't want to have all the valuable nutrients gone before the fast is even done.

Intense, Non-Stop Hunger Pains:

At times, a fast is just not meant to be. You might get halfway through and the knots in your stomach and demands for food are too much. You feel ravenously hungry and must have food. It's time to listen to your body and end the fast. Remember to use the safe exit strategy to keep from experiencing serious problems.

Hopefully, you won't have to experience any of these symptoms that lead to early termination of your fast. If you do have to stop for any reason, do the preparations and try it again. You'll make it to your goals in extended fasting if you keep trying.

9

EFFECTIVENESS OF AUTOPHAGY

HOW EFFECTIVE IS AUTOPHAGY AND DOES IT REALLY DO EVERYTHING it's touted to do? It's difficult to prove to anyone that is extra skeptical that a process happening inside the body is really happening. Autophagy does leave a few tell-tale clues that it's on the job and doing some great things. Beyond that, you have to rely on the science that's available at the moment. This chapter explores some of the definitive ways you can see autophagy at work, some of the provable benefits and where science might take things in the future.

Is Autophagy Happening?

It is hard to believe that a natural process within the body can actually be activated and stimulated to help you lose weight, rid your body of toxins, and speed up your metabolism. Yet, this is exactly what autophagy does on a daily basis. The reason you really don't notice it is because it does clean up on a small and slow scale unless encouraged by diet or cellular stress. You begin to notice a difference once the speed of autophagy increases.

Forcing Ketosis Through Diet:

One way to know that autophagy is happening is by forcing the ketosis, or fat eating process through a strict diet that virtually eliminates carbohydrates and pushes high-fat content. The only food available for the body to break down into energy is the fat. The fact that you continue to exist on a ketosis-inducing diet is proof that autophagy is happening. No single thing proves the exact amount of how much autophagy is happening in humans, but the fact that huge amounts of weight can be dropped within months shows that autophagy can get motivated with the right environment.

A huge debate rages about whether a fast is necessary if the ketosis state can be achieved through a ketogenic diet. The difference is that a water fast creates the stress state to the cells that are needed to boost the rate of autophagy. It's less about can or can't and more about how much and how fast. Sticking to a ketosis-inducing diet can add benefits for the intermittent and extended water fast. You can super-enhance the deep body cleansing and health benefits that only autophagy offers. What cannot be debated is the need for the autophagy process on a daily basis.

Life Without Autophagy:

Natural aging is a prime example of what life would be like without autophagy. It's one of the biological processes that slow down as you age. It's been discovered that rogue proteins are what unleash in the brains of the elderly and cause conditions like Parkinson's and other neurodegenerative conditions. Natural autophagy should conduct the cleaning operations it takes to isolate these proteins and recycle them or get them out of the body. Unfortunately, aging takes a toll and the autophagy process slows. Left to its own devices, you can lose your ability to detox and protect your cells.

The amount of cellular waste and "junk" doesn't decrease with age just the ability to get rid of it effectively. It could account for the higher incidences of chronic illness, cancer, leukemia, diabetes, and more in people over age 65. It's important that everyone learn how to activate and keep autophagy processes activated throughout adulthood before aging has a chance to interfere with the cleansing abilities. An important part of slowing the aging process is to invite the natural actions of the body to take a more active role on a daily basis. Part of that is by creating an environment that encourages processes like autophagy.

Why Fasting Works:

Fasting is the quickest, most direct way to add reasonable stress to the cells and trigger an autophagy response. It makes fasting one of the most effective tools available to combat the effects of aging, disease, and obesity. Fasting takes away something rather than deluging the body with chemicals and substances that may or may not work. Removing the ready-to-eat fuel forces the body to resort to cleaning and eating fat stores. The results are quick and undeniable.

Nearly anyone can do fasting, even if it's only a few hours each day, every other day, or every other week. You don't have to spend a fortune on fancy programs, equipment, or classes. All you need is a plan and a commitment to improving your health naturally. How nice would it be to spend less time at the medical center and more time out enjoying life? Imagine being able to boost your immune system to levels that you've never experienced. Autophagy can eliminate the pathogens, viruses, and bacteria that work hard to make you sick. It's a much more important physical process in the body than anyone ever dreamed.

How Soon are Changes Noticeable?

Now that you have a firm understanding of what autophagy is, why it's important, and how it' boosted, it's time to explore the time table of results. How long does it take to see real change with autophagy? Is it something that takes years to realize the complete benefits? The answer is no. You can see some changes almost immediately. Others increase over time. It's often a cumulative effect that provides the cure to our ails. The body works in harmony to get the job done.

Begin Dropping Fat Stores Right Away:

You will begin losing real pounds of fat right away when placing your body into a triggering position to increase autophagy. The ketogenic diet works, but fasting is quicker. Both offer results that are measurable on the scale. Women can lose inches of fat off their midsection in a short amount of time, even if weight loss was not their main goal. It's the midsection fat that's dangerous. It indicates you might be on the way to developing heart disease. No one can deny that autophagy is at work when you begin dropping serious pounds over a short amount of time.

You may wonder how autophagy decides to eat fat reserve cells over other tissue, such as muscles. The fact is that some tissue loss is experienced due to autophagy, but at some point, it stops and recognizes that the muscles are needed, and the fat cells are not. It's the intelligence that is innate in every fiber of the human body. In a case of actual starvation, the autophagy system would eventually have no choice but to begin eating everything in a bid to stay alive. All of the fat stores would have been exhausted at this point.

The Ketosis Exhaustion:

Another way to definitively know that autophagy is at work is the dramatic wall of exhaustion that comes down when the energy is derived from burning fat over burning carbs and sugars. You have the energy to do things, but the energy seems different somehow.

All actions are done with more purpose because it seems to require more effort. It's not a statement as to whether it's good or bad, but a notice that it's different. The first tell-tale sign that you have entered a state of ketosis is this exhaustion wall that completely envelopes you.

Immediate Improved Concentration and Memory Skills:

Fasting is shown to improve mental acuity right away. Mental acuity is your ability to focus, concentrate and remember things. Not only does autophagy run through and capture the proteins that cause neurological damage, but it also improves neuroplasticity. Every nerve and brain centered function is improved in this manner. It's the main reason why most people state that they feel they think more clearly after fasting.

Faster Recovery After Exercise:

Exercise always causes cell damage. It's the process of tearing and healing that build muscles. The recovery time after a serious workout can be a day or two but using a combination of fasting and targeted diet can minimize the recovery time. It also indicates that your healing time after an injury will speed up if you are faithful in fasting routines and using a ketosis-inducing diet. It's a simple way that shows autophagy is hard at work every day.

Relieve Inflammation Within Weeks:

Inflammation is a problem for millions of people for a variety of reasons. Some people suffer from arthritis and others have inflammation due to other chronic illnesses. Inflammation is normally due to a build-up of uric acid in the body. It tends to settle in the joints and cause stiffness, soreness, swelling and generalized irritation. Fasting and watching your diet can get rid of inflammation in a matter of weeks. It's one of the biggest selling points for fasting.

The Push for Long-Term Benefits

Scientists have designs on learning more about autophagy in humans and how it can benefit other areas of the body beyond cellular cleaning and sorting. Many of these scientists feel there are more unknown abilities to this process and the cells designated with autophagy duty. Excitement is in the air that real breakthroughs in major scientific discovery are right around the corner. Only time will tell at what will be revealed in the months and years to come. It could get interesting.

Better than a Vaccine:

What if you have instant immunity from any germ, virus, or bacteria known? What if your own autophagy cells could be trained to hunt down and kill anything that invaded your body? It could realistically be the next step up from vaccines. Your cells are specific to your DNA and can offer the best protection from a foreign invasion. It could easily outperform the current hit and miss quality of vaccinations. No adverse reactions would happen because they are your own cells. It seems like a far distant dream, but the current scientific research around genetics and gene repair is getting us closer.

It seems every day there is a new story about some mysterious disease or illness that keeps planes grounded at airports and people in quarantine. How great would it be to step outside your door and know that your own body has you protected from any pathogen out there looking for a host? Who knows what actual science it would take to promote these particular cells to super-protectors, but the idea is on the table and is getting scientists seriously interested in learning more. You could see children born in the near future that are immune to anything and everything.

Autophagy and the Fountain of Youth:

The ability for autophagy to bring a more youthful exuberance to anyone that regularly fasts and actually provides for some of the youthful qualities that cells possess, it has many scientists wondering if this might be the new fountain of youth being explored. The talk is increasingly circling around a stoppage and reversal of age using autophagy. Wouldn't it be nice to fast for a couple of days and see ten years roll off the aging clock? Could this really happen? Who knows? Apparently, almost anything under the sun is possible in this increasingly scientifically advanced universe.

Autophagy Cellular Surgery:

How wild does it sound to have a future filled with surgery-less surgery? Another thought-tasked group is studying the feasibility of cells that are responsible for the autophagy in humans to do the repair and healing from within, eliminating the need for surgery. As strange as it sounds, it would open up whole new possibilities in the world of medicine and healing. It remains to be seen if any of these ideas will prove to be viable. With the elimination of communicable diseases and surgery-less surgery, things are looking up for cheaper health insurance.

Autophagy and the Cancer Cure:

The cure for cancer has been sought since the first diagnosis. Autophagy cells have an amazing ability to inhibit the growth of cancer cells and destroy tumors. What scientists and researchers can't understand is why it isn't on a consistent basis. At times, they actually help the cancer cells thrive. If these cells could be directed always to attack and get rid of cancer cells it would be the ultimate cure. You wouldn't even have to take medications, chemotherapy, or radiation. Your cells would simply kill them off before they had a chance to be noticed. Cancer would simply fade from our memories.

10

AUTOPHAGY AND PHYSICAL FITNESS

THE ROLE PHYSICAL FITNESS PLAYS WITH AUTOPHAGY IS ONE OF BOTH enabler and benefactor. Autophagy helps ensure that you get and stay physically fit as part of a natural process. Physical fitness, in turn, can increase the amount of autophagy your body does. Physical fitness and weight management are all highly dependent on this process that keeps the cells of the body in a healthy condition. Without one, you won't have the other.

The Importance of Planning Exercise Routines and Autophagy Cycles

The mixed messages and information out there about exercise, diets, autophagy, and what should be done can get confusing. Hopefully, this chapter will clear up some of the mysteries and questions you have about physical fitness, exercise routines, and where autophagy fits into the big picture. Don't make some of the mistakes that newbie water fasters make that can jeopardize your muscle tissues.

Never Plan Intense Exercise and No Calories:

In the interest of trying to find shortcuts and cut weight more dramatically, there's a dangerous theory floating around out there that if you jump on an exercise of any sort, hit it hard, smack in the middle of a fast you'll lose tons more weight. Well, some people gave it a try and the results were not great. That mistake ends up costing you more than fat reserves. Your autophagy cells start grabbing muscle tissue as well and dining.

If you plan to exercise during the middle or at the end of a fasting period, make the activity no more than moderate, especially when it comes to cardio. The last thing you want is to have heart cells being eaten for lunch or dinner by your own body. It's critical you get the planning right for your exercise and fasting if you are a highly active person.

Without finding the right balance you can do more harm than good. Autophagy is a good thing when you keep in mind that stirring it up means it will devour almost any cell type when placed on demand of high-intensity activity and low nutrient levels.

Change Your Diet for Exercise:

Calorie restriction diets and low carbs are all the rage for dropping body fat through ketosis, but is it the right move when you are doing intense fitness workouts or training? The one thing to remember during all the rush to restrict foods and calories is to keep the protein coming. Your body needs the essential building blocks of protein to create, strengthen, and add to muscle.

You need to add carbs back into the meal before your exercise. Your body will need the fuel for energy, or it will take it from the sources you don't want to lose. Add plenty of fruits and vegetables to the menu to help replace the vital nutrients that are lost during intense exercise.

Change Your Exercise for Fasting:

You can't maintain the same level of physical activity if you are fasting and choosing ties that are too far away from your fed state. Most people don't feel energetic enough to exercise for any length of time without having nutrition to back it up. Better planning will allow you to keep the same exercise routine. You may have to switch the style of fasting you do that will allow a meal closer to your workout opportunity.

Reducing or taming your exercise routine might be the best solution for times you are fasting. It could mean reducing the days per week that you exercise. It takes compromise at times to reach the level of fasting and exercise that make you feel comfortable. The selection of intermittent fasting choices is numerous, which means there is a world of opportunities to provide for safe execution of the exercise activity you like while maintaining the fasting program you need.

The 2-Meal Rule and Water Fasting

Having the necessary nutrition to back your fasting is necessary to keep you healthy both during and after. As the name suggests, water fasting focuses on maintaining the equivalent water hydration and cuts the nutrients for designated periods of time. Attempting to keep the same strenuous exercise or physical fitness regimen while restricting nutrients is a no-no if you are eating less than 2 meals in a 24-hour period or are on a complete fast for that 24-hour time period. No exceptions exist for this rule as it has everything to do with safety for the person trying to push these boundaries.

Why 2 Meals are Necessary:

The need for protein should be a given if you are regularly partaking in physical fitness routines. The muscles undergo tearing and need the protein for repair and growth. Trying to run your engines on an empty tank won't get you very far down the road without a breakdown. It's important to remain flexible in your planning of diet, fasting, and exercise so that everything meshes well, and your health is safeguarded. Vigorous exercise at the wrong end of your fasting schedule can cause muscle loss along with fat. It cannot be over-emphasized. Never skip the proteins your body needs in the meals before and after the workout.

The meal you eat right before your workout needs to have a reduction in fats and rise in carbohydrates. The ketogenic diet pushes for increased fats and reduced carbs at all times. You need to adjust this to fit carbs in for the pre-workout meals without exception. It will help preserve your internal organ tissues that can be broken down for food by your body in extreme autophagy mode.

Stay highly aware of how you feel as you work out and fast. You will have to adjust the nutrition and activity to find your happy medium.

The Beautiful Combination of Intermittent Water Fasting and Exercise:

Intermittent water fasting seems to be perfectly matched for anyone that is involved in regular physical fitness routines or training. It is all about staying well-hydrated, which is important to anyone that stays active and fit. It's able to work with your fitness schedule by offering a huge selection of methods and programs. You can choose from alternating days, or restricted hours. You have plenty of opportunities to fit your exercise in around designated meal hours. It simplifies the planning of healthy routines and habits.

You have the opportunity to supercharge your autophagy by combining strong programs of both exercise and intermittent water fasting. Your fat burning potential will be through the roof as long as you make sure your body has enough extra carbs to draw from. You can add as strenuous and vigorous of an exercise routine as you can handle as long as you are sensible and mindful of your nutrition and meal times. Not staying on top of these details will simply throw you into starvation mode and you'll lose all types of cells from the physical activity. It can lead to damage you didn't expect or want.

Why Exercise and Strenuous Activities Are Out During Extended Water Fasting:

Anyone that has undergone a complete water fast for a long period of time understands how draining it can be. You feel completely depleted of energy the longer the fast continues. The whole purpose is to deeply cleanse the body and trigger autophagy. It's no time to begin a new exercise routine. You shouldn't even feel energized enough to do a kickboxing session. It's a time of introspection, reflection, healing, and readjustment internally. Extended fasting is a stand-alone beneficial way to get grounded and reset for better health. Everything will fall into place once you complete the long fast.

Autophagy, Exercise, and Healthy Weight Management

Autophagy has everything to do with total physical fitness and weight management. All the typical struggles with diets and fluctuating weight disappear once you have a firm grasp on the controls that determine when and why body fat is converted to energy or removed from the body. No one part is more important or less critical than another. It requires the combination of sensible diets, regular exercise, and the dependable assistance of autophagy. When all three of these work in unison, healthy weight management is a breeze. If any are out of sync, you fall back into irregular weight gains and losses.

Weight Management - More than Diet:

The cure for weight gain is always sold as some type of specialized diet. It's true that what you eat will determine the building blocks your body has to work with, but it's not the entire answer. Some diets are proven to be beneficial to maintaining a healthy weight, but they must be used in combination with other things to work as part of the answer. You need:

- Healthy, sensible diet plan
- Regular, sensible exercise plan
- Motivation to stick with both
- Flexibility to make scheduling work
- Openness to try options like water fasting

Without the motivation and desire to make a weight management system work, you'll be defeated from the start. Rarely will the elements come together for you. It's part of the process to actively seek out the mix of ingredients and make the work. Better management of weight issues is what will get you better results when stepping on the scale. How serious are you about losing that extra weight from the holidays? It will show in the results you get over time. No magic pill or potion exists, but you can use autophagy to advance progress to a degree most are unaware is possible. All done without being bound to a strict diet or calorie limitation.

How to Balance Exercise, Work, and Fasting:

Learning to balance a full work schedule and have time for healthier routines of fasting and exercise can seem frustrating. You want to do the right thing, but life seems to be getting in the way. Most of us can't do much about the work schedule. Everything else has to be fit in somewhere around those time demands. One great thing in recent years is the development of nationwide gyms that are open 24 hours a day. The fees to join and use the equipment are fairly reasonable. You even have access to a personal trainer for an extra fee.

All you'll have to do, beyond this, is decide which intermittent water fast routine works best for the schedule you have to maintain. Will it be more practical to fast on the weekends? Will you have to alternate days? Take your notebook out and make a basic chart that outlines every possible scenario, keeping in mind you need to have the exercise happen shortly after a meal for nutrition sake. A plan will begin to come together faster than you think. The perfect mix of all elements is there, even if you have to dig.

Customize Your Own Routine:

If you can't find a fasting schedule that works for you, why not customize one to suit your personal needs? As long as you are keeping safety and nutritional needs in mind, there are a million ways you can set the standard in fasting and exercise for your life. Why wait around for the perfect plan when you have the ability to create one? It doesn't need to be completely from scratch. You can switch a few things up and make it perfect for your situation, schedule, or exercise demands. You'll be ready to get started in no time.

You now have all the great information you need to get started on your path to physical fitness along with water fasting, which will raise your results of autophagy to new levels. The final chapter is important in dealing with the right way to exit fasts when you are experiencing problems. Please take the time to read this as often as necessary for your safety and well-being during any fasting activity. Your health is a priority over completing a fast.

11

HOW TO SAFELY BREAK THE AUTOPHAGY CYCLE

BEGINNING AN INTERMITTENT OR EXTENDED FAST AND HAVING TO stop for any reason must be done in a way that is safe and ultimately addresses the problem. If hunger and the need for food is the reason you are bailing on a fast, you still must be careful in what you eat to avoid calorie shocking your system. You can easily end up losing all that food with one bout of extreme nausea. Take heed to use caution and prepare an exit strategy in case it's needed at any time.

Safely Exiting the Intermittent Fast

Even though the intermittent fast isn't as grueling as the extended version, it still pays to take precautions and exit the fast safely. You should address any emergent health concerns with a doctor right away. Fasting of any sort is not agreeable with every person and every health condition. You may not even be aware of a health problem until the fast brings it to the surface. Unrecognized illnesses or bad timing can all contribute to the need to exit the fast for the time being. Below is the best way to handle the more common problems that cause an exit.

Blood Sugar Drops:

One of the more common problems recognized quickly is a drop of blood sugar levels during the fast portion. It can be problematic if it's causing difficulties while you are working. It can make you feel weak, dizzy, and slightly disoriented. Break the fast by drinking the equivalent of a glass of juice, slowly. You can continue with the fast if you feel it was a temporary thing but discontinue if the drop was enough to take you away from activity for a while.

Lowering of blood sugars during a fast is normal, but to have it bottom out or cause you to feel faint are not typical. You'll need to revisit your nutritional choices before fasting again and have your blood sugar tested by your physician. Your first meal should be juice, broth, or soft, tolerable foods.

Distractions:

Being heavily distracted or stressed can make fasting more difficult than intended. It's better to try and find a place to sit quietly and refocus. Being able to get to a calm, meditative state sometimes helps you move past blockages to continue the fasting process. If you still want to exit the fast and it hasn't been many hours, you should be able to resume a normal diet.

You need to consider changing your fasting schedule if there are distractions in the current routine. No schedule is perfect but look for one that offers the best chance of success.

Dizziness or Not Feeling Well:

Becoming ill during a fast or not realizing you are sick until you are deep into it can be aggravating. A sudden bout of dizziness could be blood sugar issues or blood pressure. Fasting lowers both. The illness could be stemming from the toxins leaving the body.

You can try drinking a small glass of juice and waiting a few minutes. Revisit how you're feeling. If you begin to perk up, the dizziness is most likely a blood sugar drop. You can make a safe judgment call on the length of time left on your fast. If you have hours to go, exit the fast. Your first meal needs to be juice, broth, soup, or other soft foods.

Give yourself a couple of days recuperation time and check your nutritional options to strengthen your body for the next fast.

Safely Exiting the Extended Fast

Exiting an extended fast carries more risk and you must be careful in doing so. Never stay in a bad fast too long. What this means is that suffering is not the intent of extended water fasting. It's meant to challenge and push your boundaries and really stage autophagy. If you find you're completely miserable, safely exit. If you experience medical situations, safely exit and seek medical advice. If you are happy and feel you've reached maximum benefit, safely exit. If you hit that hunger wall, safely exit.

Extreme Fatigue:

No words can describe the level of fatigue you will feel with your first extended fast. It's due to the level of detox taking place in your body. Years and years of built-up toxins are being removed. The longer you fast, the more you want to rest or sleep. If the exhaustion gets to be too much, safely exit. Break the fast with a glass of juice.

You need to spend an equivalent amount of time recuperating to the time you spent fasting. If you are three days in, take three days to recuperate. The first day should be all liquids at mealtimes. The second day can be fruits and soft foods. The third day you can resume your normal diet.

Medical Issues:

Do not hesitate to stop an extended fast for medical problems. Some can be serious and require immediate treatment. Call an ambulance and wait for further instruction from medical experts. Begin seeking medical advice the minute you feel something isn't right. You know your body better than anyone.

Satisfied with Present Results:

If you have followed the extended water fast to the limits you needed to see best results, congratulations! You can do a safe exit. Follow the rule of recuperation that states your recovery time should be equal to the duration of your fast. Use the liquid diet for the first day, fruits and soft foods the second, and whatever is tolerable thereafter.

Extreme Hunger:

Occasions do happen in which you reach a hunger wall that is too insurmountable to go through or around. It could be your body telling you that you've fasted enough and nutrition is needed. You can try a glass of juice and see if that perks you up a bit. You might be able to get a little more mileage. If you are still feeling the urge to stop the fast, stop.

Follow the safe exit strategy of equal recovery time for fasting time. Stick with a liquid diet the first day, no matter how ravenously hungry you feel. Choose your favorite fruits and soft foods the second recovery day. Celebrate with other foods you fancy on the following days.

How Soon to Begin A New Fast and Autophagy Cycle

Having to break a fast is disappointing, no matter which type, and for what reason. The preparation mentally and physically is an investment. It leaves you feeling like you did everything wrong, which is not the case. Some fasts will not work out, no matter how hard you try. It could be health, motivation, nutrition, or simply being in a bad mood. It's better to safely exit and try again another time. The length of duration between fasts depends on the situation around breaking the previous fast.

Starting a New Intermittent Water Fast:

A new intermittent water fast can start after a 24-hour recovery period from the last one. You might want to take a little longer if there are issues you need to sort out with your schedule, nutrition, or ensuring you don't have a medical problem. Once you are ready to start, jump in as you did before. Use the list below to see if you are ready to go:

- I am well hydrated
- I have eaten healthy foods to prepare
- I am feeling well
- I've not experienced any health issues since stopping the fast
- I'm motivated to get the fast going again

Starting a New Extended Water Fast:

Beginning a new extended fast is something that takes a great deal of thought. The first priority is your health. Make sure you have given at least two weeks devoted time to gaining strength back from the fast. If you stopped the fast due to a serious medical issue, see the section below. If you stopped for any other reason, have you discovered the problems and defined realistic solutions?

With fresh experience under your belt and knowledge of how grueling the extended fast can be, consider starting with some form of intermittent fast. Being successful with an extended fast might require building your body up to the challenge. It doesn't require following the IF for a month. Try it out for a few days and get the feel of the fasting process in a less intensive way. Use the following list to see if you are ready to start the extended water fast again:

- I understand and am prepared for the exhaustion phase
- I have someone that is available to help me
- I feel healthy and well
- I haven't experienced any health problems since leaving the last fast
- I'll monitor how I feel closely

Discussing Whether Fasting is Possible:

Not completing the extended fast for serious health issues is not a fun way to end things. Have an open and honest discussion with your doctor about whether you're healthy enough for long fasting. It's not an activity everyone can do safely. Find out if you can do shorter fasting or if it's an activity that is not in the best interest of your health. No shame is involved in trying to better your health and not being able to complete the program. You are an amazing person for giving it a try. Remember, there are other ways to increase autophagy!

Give These a Try if You Can't Fast:

Low-Carbohydrate Diet –

Switch to a low-carb or keto-type diet. You will probably increase autophagy. It may not get to the pace of fasting levels, but it's a safe way for you to get the benefits of autophagy when you can't safely fast. Feeling better will also happen if you drop the sugary foods, drinks, and processed items out of your diet.

30-Minute Cardio Exercises –

It doesn't require hours and hours of exercise to get the full bene-fits of autophagy. Short, intense cardio workouts do more to promote autophagy than anything else. It's worth 30-minutes out of your day to massively improve your health. It will make you feel younger for longer.

CONCLUSION

Thank you for making it through to the end of *Autophagy for Women*. Let's hope it was informative and able to provide you with all of the tools you need to achieve your goals, whatever they may be.

Autophagy is a natural process that happens at the cellular level of every human. You now know how it's connected to the system that holds the keys to metabolic processes in the body. It can help determine whether pathogens are left lurking that can make you sick, whether dead or dying cells need to be removed, or the area needs a general tidy. The cleaner autophagy can leave the environment your cells live in, the fewer your concerns will be about sudden illness, disease, rapid aging, or cancerous growths.

It's the little changes you make today that will impact you the most in the years to come. Making the commitment to better your health through autophagy will require exploring what you think the best methods are for your lifestyle, schedule, and concerns. You may not be worried about the effects of aging at 25, but it's a big deal when you're pushing 50. Alternately, at 50, most women aren't worried about reproductive health, yet a woman at 25 will find it important. Autophagy can improve the health and function of the body at the cellular level for any age.

Start in smaller ways, such as changing up your diet to encourage autophagy. Once you feel comfortable, try dabbling with the intermittent water fast. It's something you can do at your own pace and never feel guilty about not fully completing. You might find that the challenge of it becomes addicting. Intermittent fasting is not like dieting in any way. It's simply setting up periods of food deprivation. Nothing more, nothing less. It's worth a try if it can boost your autophagy potential.

Move on to the extended water fast after you've gained a good foothold on the intermittent fast. Moving too quickly can set you up for failure and disappointment. It's important to stay aware of your health, no matter which fast you try. If fasting doesn't work out for you, fall back and use the keto diet. Either way, you'll have an increased level of autophagy that is steadily working to improve your health.

You now have the knowledge in your hands and power to make some changes that could improve your life and health in ways that are astounding. You can reach deep to the cellular levels of your body and provide the cleanest, most robust help for your cells that encourages consistent, youthful performance.

Finally, if you found this book useful in any way, a review is always appreciated!

www.ingramcontent.com/pod-product-compliance
Lightning Source LLC
Chambersburg PA
CBHW031336290526
45784CB00015B/2958